extra lean
FAMILY

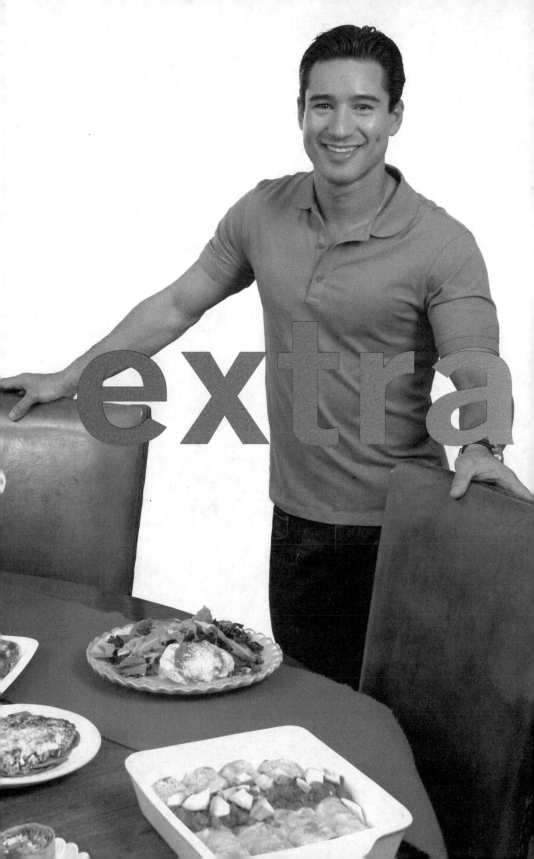

MARIO LOPEZ

with JIMMY PEÑA

lean
FAMILY

**GET LEAN AND ACHIEVE YOUR
FAMILY'S BEST HEALTH EVER**

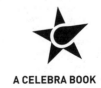

A CELEBRA BOOK

Celebra
Published by New American Library, a division of
Penguin Group (USA) Inc., 375 Hudson Street,
New York, New York 10014, USA
Penguin Group (Canada), 90 Eglinton Avenue East, Suite 700, Toronto,
Ontario M4P 2Y3, Canada (a division of Pearson Penguin Canada Inc.)
Penguin Books Ltd., 80 Strand, London WC2R 0RL, England
Penguin Ireland, 25 St. Stephen's Green, Dublin 2,
Ireland (a division of Penguin Books Ltd.)
Penguin Group (Australia), 250 Camberwell Road, Camberwell, Victoria 3124,
Australia (a division of Pearson Australia Group Pty. Ltd.)
Penguin Books India Pvt. Ltd., 11 Community Centre, Panchsheel Park,
New Delhi - 110 017, India
Penguin Group (NZ), 67 Apollo Drive, Rosedale, Auckland 0632,
New Zealand (a division of Pearson New Zealand Ltd.)
Penguin Books (South Africa) (Pty.) Ltd., 24 Sturdee Avenue,
Rosebank, Johannesburg 2196, South Africa

Penguin Books Ltd., Registered Offices:
80 Strand, London WC2R 0RL, England

Published by Celebra, a division of Penguin Group (USA) Inc. Previously published in a Celebra hardcover edition.

First Celebra Trade Paperback Printing, May 2012
10 9 8 7 6 5 4 3 2 1

Photography: Michael Darter
Food styling: Food Crew—Jeff Parker and Lisa Barnet

CELEBRA and logo are trademarks of Penguin Group (USA) Inc.

Celebra trade paperback ISBN: 978-0-451-23652-4

The Library of Congress has catalogued the hardcover edition of this title as follows:
Lopez, Mario, 1973–.
Extra lean family: get lean and achieve your family's best health ever/Mario Lopez, with Jimmy Peña.
    p. cm.
ISBN 978-0-451-23412-4
1. Weight loss. 2. Nutrition. 3. Energy metabolism. 4. Lopez family—Health.
I. Peña, Jimmy. II. Title.
RM22.2.L5758 2011
613.2′5—dc22   2010053460

Set in Din
Designed by Pauline Neuwirth

Printed in the United States of America

PUBLISHER'S NOTE
The recipes contained in this book are to be followed exactly as written. The publisher is not responsible for
your specific health or allergy needs that may require medical supervision. The publisher is not responsible for
any adverse reactions to the recipes contained in this book.
    While the authors have made every effort to provide accurate telephone numbers and Internet addresses
at the time of publication, neither the publisher nor the authors assume any responsibility for errors, or for
changes that occur after publication. Further, publisher does not have any control over and does not assume
any responsibility for author or third-party Web sites or their content.

To the most important women in my life—
Mom, Marissa, Mazza, and Gia Francesca—
for teaching me everything I know about food and love.

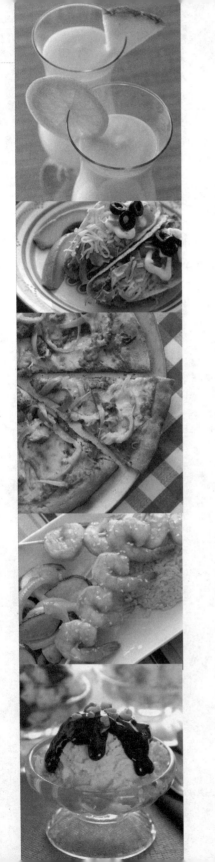

contents

extra lean
FAMILY

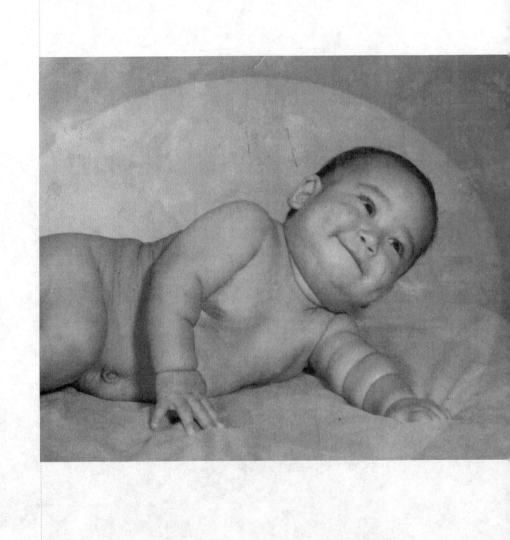

introduction

YOU CARE ABOUT your family and you want them to be healthy, energetic, and live life to the fullest.

That's what *Extra Lean Family* is all about.

My last book, *Extra Lean*, introduced a foolproof plan that radically changes the way you eat. That plan revolves around three simple yet effective rules designed to turn your body into a fat-burning machine: 1) balance your daily intake of carbs, protein, and fat; 2) practice proper portion control; and 3) eat frequently throughout the day. *Extra Lean* teaches you how to eat the right balance of foods, at just the right times and in the correct portions, to achieve a healthy weight by burning unwanted fat and calories more efficiently. Following this lifestyle even allows you to indulge occasionally without sabotaging your diet or gaining weight. You no longer feel inclined to binge on holidays or weekends, because you already eat the foods you love.

Although I live by the principles of *Extra Lean* every day, I wasn't raised on them. In fact, I was an overweight baby and basically looked like a mini version of the Michelin tire man. But the story of how I got so big is actually not based on the fact that I was gaining too much weight early on. Instead, my initial problem was that I was losing weight! To make matters worse, the doctors had no idea why and what was causing this rapid weight loss. Their only diagnosis was a "failure to thrive." My parents were so convinced that I might not make it, a priest even came in to bless me.

In desperation, my terrified father drove me south of the border to seek out a Mexican *bruja*—that's a sort of witch doctor—to help bring me back to good health. This woman mixed up some sort of concoction from different herbs and liquids. To this day, I still don't know what it was. Unbelievable as this may sound, her magical brew worked! I started gaining weight right away. Pretty soon I had huge rolls of fat all over my body—a sure sign of a healthy baby in my mother's loving eyes! She still loves to tease me about how she used to have to separate the folds of skin with her fingers to bathe me, because I was such a big baby.

As I grew into childhood, I kept eating for pleasure and developed a real passion for food. I ate everything from Mexican favorites like my grandmother's enchiladas to my mom's meatloaf and her favorite pasta dishes. My parents taught me to love food, but my Mexican upbringing meant that I didn't necessarily eat the healthiest foods I could. Luckily, my mother realized that I was the kind of child who needs lots of activities to burn off energy. As I started elementary school, she began signing me up for activities at the Boys and Girls Club. It was through this organization that I got into wrestling and other sports, and my mentors were always involved in helping me take joy in being physical and competitive. By high school, I was a wrestling champion and much more conscious of eating healthy foods for energy instead of just devouring whatever was around. As an actor, too, I realized that being fit was part of my profession. I had to look and feel good to get new roles and succeed at the challenges presented to me.

By about age eighteen, I had my own apartment and finally started cooking for myself. I was big on breakfast foods. I made scrambled eggs and put everything I had in the refrigerator into those eggs, from vegetables to cheese. I was a fan of the grill too, and grilled pretty much everything I ate for supper: fish, steaks, pork chops, and even grilled cheese.

The problem was that, because I was so busy and so anxious about being less fit than I could be, I stuck to the same boring routine of eggs, lean meats, and vegetables. In a way, I still struggled to find that balance between enjoying food and staying in shape. When it came down to it, I didn't want to sacrifice the food I loved to look good. As I learned more about my body and nutrition, I realized that by keeping my metabolism running at a maximum efficiency, calories kept coming off. And the key wasn't necessarily exercise; it was food. When I incorporated optimal combinations of daily nutrients, watched my portion sizes, and ate frequent small meals, my body was in a constant state of burning fat. As long as I followed these principles, I was able to enjoy all kinds of food without ever feeling guilty. My approach to food changed my life. I was living *Extra Lean*.

My parents taught me to love food

The same year that *Extra Lean* was published, I became a father. As I held my beautiful daughter, Gia Francesca, for the first time, I understood that every life choice I make from now on will affect my child. Children look to the people who care for them to find their way in the world. And, because children learn more from the example their parents set than from any lecture we could ever deliver, it's up to us to be the best role models possible.

When it comes to my child's health, I've realized that there's no better place for me to be a good role model than in my own family's kitchen. I've been learning that lesson all of my life. I've been blessed with a great family. The thing is, even when you come from a wonderful family like mine, you still don't fully grasp what it means to be a parent. When you're about to have a baby, everyone talks to you about what a big adjustment you'll have to make, how little sleep you'll get, and how hard you'll have to work to provide for your family. What they could never describe, which you have to experience for yourself, are the new and overwhelming emotions you'll feel that you never felt before.

When I started thinking about how I could be the best possible dad to Gia Francesca, I immediately thought of how hard my parents worked to provide for us. My parents were willing to make personal sacrifices and go to almost any lengths to help my sister and me thrive. But no matter what life threw at us, the kitchen was always the heart of our home, and my mother always made sure that there was plenty of good food on the table. In our household, food was a source of happiness.

There's no better place for me to be a good role model than in my own family's kitchen.

I want my Gia Francesca to feel that same love in the kitchen that I did and learn that food can bring both happiness and health. The kitchen is where good health starts, because it's where we prepare the food our families will eat and where we teach our kids the nutritional knowledge and attitude toward food that they will carry with them for a lifetime. This is a big responsibility and, if we don't do it right, the health risks for our children can be monumental.

Today in the United States, we're slowly killing ourselves and our families with food. Obesity is a true epidemic in our country, affecting a third of adults and nearly 20 percent of children ages six to eleven. Weight-related illnesses like diabetes and heart problems may be killing more people today, and our children are the ones who are suffering most. Research shows that overweight children are likely to grow up to become obese adults with increased health problems. This is the first generation in which our children may face a diminished life-expectancy rate because they eat the wrong foods—and too much of them.

These are scary statistics. No doubt you've already heard them. Maybe, though, you inevitably put them out of your mind, because just like millions of other people, you've developed habits and a routine that are hard to shake. Perhaps you've tried dieting but swung back again. You hardly have time to get everyone out the door in the morning, never mind think about planning healthier menus. Plus, you look at the huge portions in restaurants, the types of foods served in school cafeterias, and the way your kids gorge themselves on fried foods and sugary snacks at friends' houses, and feel that it's too hard to control what your family eats.

For me, living *Extra Lean* has allowed me to control my health and body while enjoying the foods I love. I want the same for my family. The core purpose of *Extra Lean Family* is taking the basic principles for the individual from *Extra Lean* and applying them to the household. On a group level, I've learned that the most effective way to instill the *Extra Lean* principles and change the way you and your family eat is to follow three crucial steps:

1. Understand *Extra Lean Family*
2. Prepare *Extra Lean Family*
3. Maintain *Extra Lean Family*

The first focuses on how changing the way your family eats requires a basic understanding of metabolism. This is how I first came to discover the *Extra Lean* principles and this is how you and your family can live *Extra Lean*. Learn how to make your metabolism work for you through specific, fat-burning foods, proper portion control, and frequent meals. This step creates a foundation for your family to absorb all the nutrition and weight loss information you'll ever really need to keep your metabolisms running high for life.

The second step ensures that each member of your family and household is prepared to apply the *Extra Lean* principles and transition into healthy eating. Through tangible methods that everyone can do together, this step teaches your family how to evaluate the foods you eat on a regular basis and change the state of your home and habits to help you achieve a new approach to food and eating.

The third teaches the family how to maintain this new approach to food and lean living while on the meal plan and beyond. While changing your family's eating habits sounds daunting enough, what's more challenging is maintaining your focus while going through the routine of everyday life. Most people want to eat well but hectic schedules and time conflicts can get in the way of good intentions. This third step teaches your family how to prep ahead of time and plan your meals in advance so that the main focus will always be eating good foods that will boost your metabolism.

And finally, the five-week plan was designed to implement these three steps so that you can truly experience living *Extra Lean* as a family every day. Here, you'll find meals that are quick, healthy, and delicious. The key strength of the meals is that it shows you how to combine nutrients in the right proportions for your family to stay satisfied while keeping off unnecessary weight. That's because the daily intake of nutrients is set in the general fat-burning proportions of 50% carbs, 25% protein, and 25% healthy fats. The meal plan also includes all of these easy components and guidelines to help you and your family reach your health goals:

>> Simple, delicious recipes that can be prepared in twenty minutes or less
>> Double Duty meal options to satisfy different taste buds and moods by offering two quick variations using the same main ingredients
>> Prep tips and advice to help you plan ahead for the coming week
>> A generous list of simple, filling, nutritious snacks to combat hunger between meals and keep everyone's metabolism moving at optimum speed
>> Detailed food planning tools, like shopping lists, ways to prepare and freeze meals ahead, and information about how to turn leftovers into quick and satisfying meals

Taken together, the many tools and resources in *Extra Lean Family* will teach you how to become a great role model for your family in the kitchen and at the dinner table, as you help the people you love most achieve their best health for a lifetime.

One of the most important life lessons my mother taught me was this: "There's no such thing as a shortcut."

When it comes to making a lifestyle shift as major as changing how and what your family eats, that's a lesson worth remembering. It took me many years, and several false starts, to transform my attitude toward food. I hope that by passing on my principles for living *Extra Lean*, you and your family will have a reason to start your new approach to food and healthy living. By using this book, you will explore a whole new world of different, nutritious foods and, because the recipes are so quick and easy, you'll have more family time, too. Most importantly, you'll come away with the foundation you need to help you and your children avoid the body issues and health risks that plague so many Americans.

The kitchen was always the heart of our home.

As someone who has enjoyed learning about fitness and food for himself, and as a new father who is dedicated to raising his daughter to be as healthy and happy as possible, I am passionate about passing on my love for food to those I love the most. Good health for your family starts at home, right in your own kitchen. Make yourself the best role model your child will ever have when it comes to reaching your family's short- and long-term health goals and live life to the fullest.

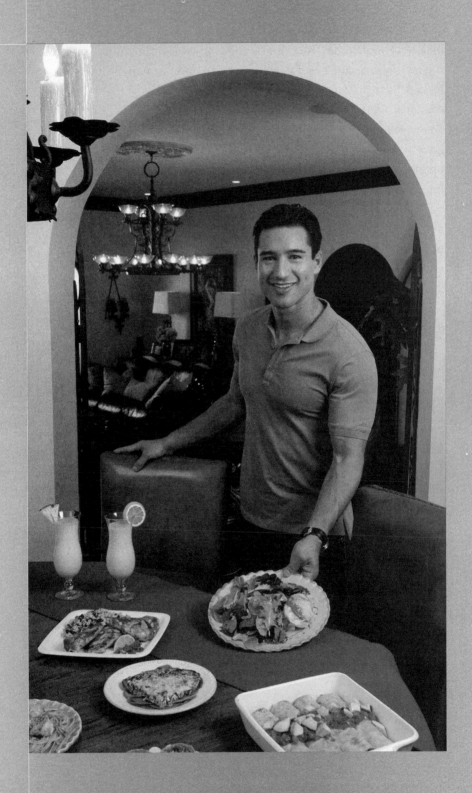

understand
extra lean family

To KNOW WHAT it means to be an *Extra Lean Family*, you'll need to learn these three simple yet effective steps: 1) understand your metabolism, 2) follow the ten nutrition rules to boost your metabolism, and 3) know what a healthy plate looks like. These steps ensure that what you know and do each and every day will contribute to an efficient metabolism for life.

The first step teaches you that the most basic thing to learn is your own body's metabolism—the process your body goes through to break down food to get energy—and that only you can control how the metabolism works for the body.

Step Two is all about grasping the ten simple nutrition rules to boost your metabolism. Read these rules, and make them your own. By doing so, you'll soon discover that your body has the ability to burn off calories and fat efficiently—even when you're not doing anything more active than driving your car or sitting on the couch!

Finally, in Step Three, you will learn foolproof strategies to practice good portion control, which is the most effective way to keep your metabolism high without sacrificing the foods you love. Even the very youngest members of your family can learn what a healthy plate looks like, with the right balance of carbs, protein, and fat in just the right amounts for each of you to feel maximum energy while absorbing a minimum of unnecessary calories.

Follow these steps to optimize your metabolism and maintain your ideal weight while eating healthy, quick, delicious meals and snacks.

STEP 1: Understanding Your Metabolism

"Metabolism" is shorthand for that complex chemical dance inside your body among your brain, your gut, your hormones, and your body's fat cells, as they all work together to determine how quickly or how slowly your body burns fuel. *Extra Lean* was founded on the principle that you can control your metabolism and train your body to constantly burn fat just by following three simple rules when it comes to what you eat, how much you eat, and how many times you eat: 1) balance your daily intake of carbs, protein, and fat; 2) practice proper portion control; and 3) eat frequently throughout the day. These are the only principles you will need to maintain a healthy weight and lean body because each is a crucial factor to achieve an efficient metabolism.

The first step teaches you how to balance the three basic macronutrients—carbs, protein, and fat—essential for your body to function properly. When you fuel your body with the right amounts of these nutrients, you create the optimal state that allows every function of your body to perform its best, namely your metabolism.

The second step then trains you to eat the balance of foods in the right amounts. You and your family each need enough calories and nutrients to give you the energy you need—not too much, and not too little—for your metabolism to be at its most efficient. Practicing proper portion control will ensure that you don't consume excess amounts of calories, which can definitely lead to weight gain and ultimately decrease the performance of your metabolism.

The third step allows your metabolism to efficiently convert calories to energy by eating the right amounts of nutrient-dense food throughout the day. I like to compare a body's metabolism to a fire in a furnace. If you throw a huge log on that fire, it'll be tough for it to burn. However, if you feed smaller pieces of wood into the furnace, you'll see that the wood is being consumed much more efficiently. This is the way your body works when you eat frequently throughout the day.

The three principles of *Extra Lean* show the crucial role that food plays in keeping your metabolism high. On the other hand, if you starve yourself and hold back on the fuel you need, your body will start shutting down to conserve energy. That's bound to reduce your metabolism to just a flicker, and you won't have the energy you need to achieve your best health. The meals in *Extra Lean Family* are specifically designed to keep your metabolism high because your daily meals will have the proper balance of carbs, protein, and fat in the right portions and amounts.

Food is just one thing that influences your metabolism. Your body composition has a lot to do with your metabolic rate—the amount of muscle and fat you have on your body. The more muscle or lean tissue you have, the higher your metabolism will be. That's because our muscle cells burn through more calories at rest than our fat cells do, so the more fat you have, the fewer calories your body will burn at rest.

Ideally, you want to get your metabolism to the point where the foods you eat and the composition of your body are such that you burn a high amount of calories even when you're sitting still. The better fueled and productive you are *for* activity, the more fat you'll burn when doing virtually nothing.

You can boost your metabolism by eating just the right quantity and combination of foods, as the meals and snacks are laid out in *Extra Lean Family*. Once you combine these two factors, your body will be a constant fat-burning machine, allowing you to enjoy food more than ever as you achieve your best health.

EXTRA LEAN KIDS

WHEN IT COMES to your kids, chances are that metabolism isn't a huge issue right now. The human body's metabolism typically doesn't start slowing down until our twenties. I definitely feel like my own metabolism has changed. As a teenager playing sports, I used to be able to come home after practice and eat a dozen tacos followed by a pint of ice cream without gaining an ounce. That's certainly not true anymore. The reason you want to make your child aware of healthy eating habits now is so that she can maintain a healthy metabolism into adulthood. You want to teach your children that it's important to have those small, frequent, nutritious meals during the day, so that they'll learn to have healthy snacks not just at home, but when they go to school, play sports, and visit friends.

STEP 2: Follow the Top Ten Nutrition Rules to Boost Your Metabolism

I enjoy food without guilt. I'm definitely one of those people who lives to eat. I want you and your family to do the same. With the delicious and wholesome meals in *Extra Lean Family*, your diet won't be limited. In fact, you will explore a wide variety of foods to ensure that you receive the benefits of as many nutrients as possible.

By the time you finish the plan, you'll think of food as your friend, not your enemy, because food provides the fuel for your body and energy throughout the day.

This step encompasses the top ten nutrition rules that I live by to boost my metabolism. I didn't think of these rules overnight. This knowledge came to me gradually, first as a teenager who started reading about nutrition and fitness and testing out different ways of eating on my own. Later, as I hit my mid-twenties, a lightbulb went off as I realized that it was going to take more work on my part to dial back the quantity and types of food I was eating if I wanted to avoid potential weight gain. Working out just wasn't cutting it anymore when it came to staying lean. Believe me, TV really does add pounds, so it was easy for me to see when

I was doing something right and when I was doing something wrong as far as my eating habits were concerned. I knew I had to look at food in a whole new way.

I also developed my own nutrition rules because I didn't like any of the popular diets being advertised or tried—and abandoned—by so many people. I knew myself well enough to know that I'd be really miserable if I had to give up my favorite foods. I'm just not the type of person who would be able to consistently live on just grapefruit for breakfast, for instance, or to eliminate carbs completely from my diet. My goal, which I began to accomplish in creating the *Extra Lean* plan and have been refining since for my own family, was to create a plan that would allow me and anyone else, of any age, to enjoy a wide variety of healthy foods designed to keep your body's metabolism in prime shape.

1. EAT AT LEAST FIVE TIMES A DAY

If you have a family, then you know that most children don't want to sit for three big meals a day. Kids would rather graze. Two hours after lunch, and there they are again, rooting around in the kitchen for a snack.

Some parents might react to this as a sign of overeating and discourage eating frequently to prevent heavy consequences down the road. This is a knee-jerk response because most of us were raised to think that sitting down to three meals a day is the healthiest way to eat. But, in fact, kids have it right after all: the human body is most energy efficient if it's fueled by smaller meals eaten more frequently throughout the day. Due to proven results, nutrition experts now agree that eating five to seven times *every day* is far more effective in terms of keeping your metabolism running high. I grazed when I was a kid, eating all day long, and I still do it today, because I know it's absolutely the healthiest thing I can do for my body.

If you restrict yourself to eating only three times a day, you will probably gobble down larger portion sizes (and many more calories) because you feel so hungry. How many times have you sat down with a friend for lunch and heard her say, "Wow! I'm starving!"

You don't want to let your body get to that point. Think about it: If your family eats breakfast at seven a.m., lunch at noon, and dinner at six p.m., that's between five and six hours between meals. It's no wonder that some people end up coming home from school or work, reaching into the pantry, and gobbling down cereal, chips, and cookies the minute they step in the door! You're far better off eating *before* you get really hungry.

Also, the human body is at its most efficient if you eat only a certain amount of nutrients at each sitting. Every time you eat, your metabolism increases, and the higher your metabolism, the more body fat you'll burn. Eating frequently means that your metabolism will be raised that many more times than when eating just three times a day. Plus, since you're eating every two or three hours, your metabolism won't have time to slow down. You'll be burning fat all day long and you'll weigh less and have more energy.

2. AVOID EMPTY CALORIES

If I have a handful of chips when I'm running between meetings and can't stop for a meal or a nutritious snack, I feel terrible. Experience has taught me that if I eat trail mix or a protein bar when I'm on the go, I have the energy I need to get things done. That's why I usually keep a bag of healthy snacks in my car, so that if I'm stuck in traffic or don't have time to stop between leaving work and making it home, I can keep my metabolism going strong.

One key rule of mine is never eat empty calories. Don't frequently eat just anything. Make sure that you consume foods with a nutritional punch at each sitting. Those sugary cereals, fatty fried foods, and plain pastas, for instance, are just empty calories—that is, you're getting a lot of calories but very little nutrition, which means that your body will store those extra empty calories as body fat instead of burning them as fuel.

3. SEEK VARIETY

Growing up, I ate the foods I loved—again and again. I found a few meals that were healthy and helped me stay in shape, and I ate them every single day. For example, I always had eggs for breakfast, tuna fish

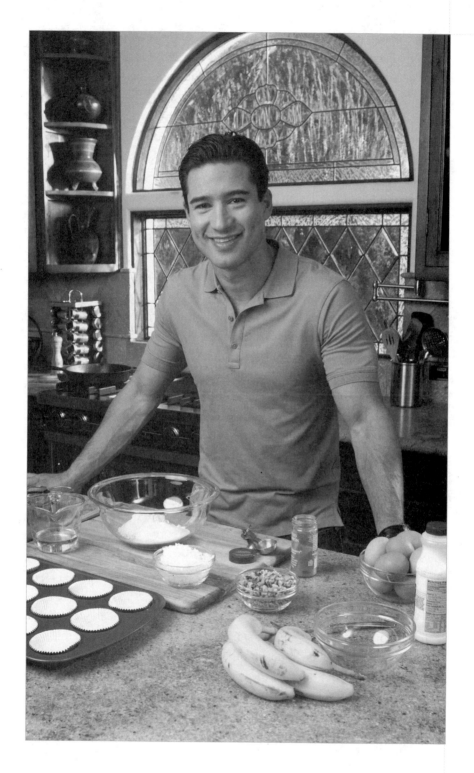

or a chicken breast with broccoli at lunch, and a lean piece of meat for dinner. Even my snacks were made up of the same foods!

For busy families, it's easy to fall into the same sort of rut I did. You rush to the grocery store without a list, so you buy the same items you bought last time, simply because you carry the recipes in your head. Or maybe you waver between making one of your usual dinners and another, more exciting meal, then decide to make the same meal the kids liked last time. Why cook something the kids won't eat, right? And why make things harder on yourself?

The problem with this pattern is that human beings love variety. We're curious animals, and if we don't feed our natural culinary curiosity one way, we'll feed it another—by snacking on unhealthy foods or eating our favorite dessert, for instance, because we lack diversity and excitement in our meals and snacks.

In addition to getting bored, we are also depriving ourselves of essential nutrients if we eat the same foods. Every food has its own individual nutrient profile, with different amino acids (the building blocks of proteins), carbohydrates, fats, vitamins, and minerals. To boost your health and energy, you need all of those different nutrients. No one food can provide your body with everything it needs. For that matter, no combination of ten or even twenty different foods will do that.

In the five-week plan, you'll find all kinds of different meats, vegetables, grains, fruits, and dairy items popping up. I want every family to experience a wide variety of foods to ensure that everyone absorbs every beneficial nutrient imaginable. And who knows? Your picky toddler or teen might even discover a new favorite taste!

4. POWER UP WITH PROTEIN

It's no secret among my friends and family that I eat lean steaks and chicken breasts on a regular basis. That's because I've learned through experience that protein keeps me from feeling hungry and gives me the energy I need to get through my workday—and to do my best workouts, too. Low fat cuts of meat, poultry, and fish are incredible sources of high-quality protein. Most importantly, these are considered complete proteins, which provide all of the essential elements of protein your body needs. Just be sure to choose healthy cooking methods, which include broiling, boiling, grilling, poaching, or roasting—avoid deep-frying meat or adding unnecessary fats when you cook.

Milk and dairy products are great for adding protein to your family's diet, too. When I was a kid, I drank five or six glasses of whole milk a day. Now, of course, I've switched to nonfat milk and yogurt, and so should you. Make the transition gradually, using 2 percent and 1 percent first before you buy skim or nonfat products. That way, your family will adapt more easily.

I grew up eating my mom's homemade Mexican food, and beans came in just about everything and with everything, from enchiladas to chili and stews. Beans are one of the best ways to give your family a great daily dose of protein for much less money than meat. Beans are high in fiber, too, and low in cholesterol. Just try to avoid making them the way my grandmother did—she loved to put lard in her beans to add flavor while she cooked

BEST SOURCES OF
lean protein

- ▶ Beans (avoid beans that are cooked with fats or sugars)
- ▶ Chicken or turkey breast (always take off the skin and trim the fat)
- ▶ Tofu (this is a nicely versatile protein source because it takes on the flavor of whatever you cook with it)
- ▶ Lean cuts of beef and pork (choose round steaks and roast for beef, tenderloin and center loin for pork)
- ▶ Shrimp
- ▶ Cod, mahi mahi, tilapia, or any other mild white fish
- ▶ Whole grains
- ▶ Eggs
- ▶ Dairy products such as nonfat yogurt, milk, and cheese

them. They were definitely delicious, but about as fattening a food as you can get! Luckily, it's easy to season beans to give them flavor without adding all of those unnecessary calories. You'll find lots of recipes for beans in the meal plan that will show you some great ways to make the most of this age-old source of protein.

Now that I'm an adult, I've come to appreciate the wonders of tofu as another good, low-cost source of lean protein. Tofu is low in calories but leaves you feeling satisfied. Just don't go for the deep-fried tofu. Instead, try it with a low sodium marinade stir-fried in with veggies. You can find tofu in the meals in this book because of the nutritional benefits and the versatility in preparation. Don't let your kids talk you out of trying them! I wish I'd discovered tofu earlier in my life.

When considering what you want to spend your calories on, ideally your daily calories will consist of 25 percent to 30 percent protein if you're an adult. For children and teens, 20 percent of their daily intake should be protein. This will allow everyone in the family to maintain lean muscle, boost metabolism high to keep calories coming off, and sidestep food cravings that may derail your overall eating habits and health.

5. FOCUS ON THE RIGHT FATS

Just hearing the word "fat" probably makes you wince. Whether or not you're overweight, you've probably come to believe that fat is bad for you. Quite the opposite is true. Just like protein, fats are key players when it comes to gearing your body up to maximum efficiency. Fats help you produce hormones, regulate temperature, absorb important fat-soluble vitamins like A, D, E and K, and build up shock absorption in your joints. Fats even help your nervous system function properly. And, like carbohydrates, which I'll discuss in a minute, fats provide important, long-lasting fuel for your body to burn during intense exercise.

The biggest surprise for me, as I started learning about food, is that eating *the right kinds of fat in the right amounts* isn't just good for your health, it's also the best way to lose weight more easily. I know a lot of people who can't believe that I eat nuts to stay lean, because of the amount of fat in nuts. But eating nuts will give you omega-3 fatty acids, which are essential for healthy body functions, and that handful of almonds you eat as a snack may actually help you lose weight. That's because it takes your body more time to digest fat than carbohydrates, so you're left feeling more satisfied and have longer-lasting energy after a meal.

THE BATTLE BETWEEN "BAD" AND "GOOD" FATS

I love to cook with olive oil and I regularly eat eggs for breakfast. That may surprise you, if you've grown up thinking that you can't lose weight if you eat fat. But the recipes in *Extra Lean Family* are packed with healthy fats to make the food taste great, keep you satisfied, and boost your family's health at the same time.

The bottom line is that your body needs fat. As I will continue to emphasize, about 25 percent to 30 percent of your daily calories should come from fat—and that's especially true if you want to lose weight.

On television and in magazines, you've probably heard discussions about how some fats are "good" and others are "bad." The "bad" fats are defined by nutrition experts as trans fats or saturated fats. What's the difference? If a fat's a fat, it's still bad for you, right?

Wrong. It's the type of fat you consume, not the total amount of fat, that may up your risk of developing heart disease. The worst culprits? Trans fats (hydrogenated oil) and saturated fats (found in meats and dairy).

Trans fats have really moved onto the nation's health radar lately, and it's a good thing. When vegetable oil is turned into a solid, it has the same effect on your body as butter. Although some trans fatty acids are found naturally in small quantities in some foods, like beef, butter, and milk, most of the trans fats (short for "trans fatty acids") we've been eating have been man-made. A lot of the ready-to-eat packaged foods you see on your supermarket shelves—almost half, in fact—contain trans fats, including crackers, granola bars, chips, and other snack foods. That's why it's so important to read food labels when you shop.

Trans fats and saturated fat both raise the level of LDL cholesterol in your arteries—not a good thing, since that buildup can lead to clogged arteries and increase the risk of stroke or heart attack. Even worse, trans fats cause HDL cholesterol levels—that's the good kind of cholesterol

continued

because it helps your body stream waste products out of your arteries and to your liver—to go down.

Making sure that your family's diet includes those "good" fats, the unsaturated fats that keep cholesterol low, will help your family stay healthy. The two main types of unsaturated fats are MUFAs (monounsaturated fatty acids) and PUFAs (polyunsaturated fatty acids). Foods high in MUFAs include olive oil, canola oil, avocados, and peanut butter. Look to salmon, safflower oil, walnuts, and sunflower seeds if you want to boost your PUFAs.

When you start using the *Extra Lean Family* plan, it will become easy for you to see how to add more of these MUFAs and PUFAs to your family's meals. You'll find snacks and sandwiches with peanut butter, avocados in salads, main dishes with salmon, and olive oil in many of the dishes, because I want you to see how easy it is to boost your good cholesterol levels.

Why the bad rap, then? Notice that I said *the right kinds of fats in the right amounts.* The thing about all fats is that they provide a more concentrated source of calories. Two grams of protein and two grams of carbs each give you eight calories, for instance, but two grams of fat will probably give you double that. You want to eat maybe ten almonds for a snack, but don't polish off the whole bag! Portion control and eating foods in the right balance are key to reaching and maintaining a healthy weight.

THOSE AWESOME OMEGAS

Spinach is a great source of omega-3 fatty acid. So are mangoes, which I love to blend with nonfat vanilla yogurt for a great smoothie that can serve as my breakfast on a hectic morning or a great nutritious snack between meals. Omega-3 and omega-6 fatty acids pack a big nutritional punch, especially for children and teens, because these polyunsaturated fats (PUFAs) boost growth and brain function. Like all PUFAs, they also reduce the risk of heart disease and stroke by lowering cholesterol. Your body can't produce either of these special fats on its own, so it's important to fit them into your family's diet.

BEST SOURCES OF
omega-3 **fats:**
► Fish like salmon, tuna, sardines, and anchovies
► Flaxseeds
► Walnuts
► Soybeans
► Wheat germ

BEST SOURCES OF
omega-6 **fats:**
► Soy
► Meat
► Poultry
► Eggs
► Nuts
► Seeds

6. GET CLUED INTO CARBOHYDRATES

Just a quick glance into the windows of the cars around you when you're driving to work or school should be evidence enough that we live in a world where most people rely on carbohydrates for fuel: there's a woman drinking a soda, a man eating a candy bar, kids snacking on cookies and chips in the backseat.

I'm no exception. I grew up eating my grandmother's homemade tortillas. After school, I'd come into the kitchen and warm them up on the stove, get a stick of butter, and rub the tortillas all over with butter. I'd eat six or seven tortillas without even sitting down.

Why do we crave starchy, sugary foods like tortillas, pasta, potatoes, cakes, and other so-called comfort foods that are all carbohydrates?

Because carbohydrates—"carbs" for short—are the human body's preferred energy source for mind and body. Your brain, especially, relies on carbs to function, which is why following diets that restrict your carb intake make you feel like you can't think straight. My rule of thumb is to never, ever skimp on carbs. In *Extra Lean*, I showed that all major meals should be composed of at least 50 percent carbs. The same applies to the meals in *Extra Lean Family*. Carbs are especially essential for active kids who are growing fast and playing sports.

A lot of people go on fad diets that ask them to give up carbohydrates altogether. They usually can't stick to them—or find that they start feeling like they're low on energy. What happens to your body if you don't get enough carbs? It stops working efficiently and you'll feel drained of energy, too, as your body resorts to releasing previously stored carbs or tries to convert other macronutrients into carbs to keep you going. Many people have the misconception that eating carbs will make you fat, but that's not necessarily true. When you eat the right kinds of carbs and in the right amounts, they can actually do the opposite and help you lose weight.

How do you get clued into the right carbs, so that you and your family can enjoy good food without guilt? It's important to know that there are two main categories of carbohydrates: simple and complex. Simple carbs from foods like fruits and vegetables are quickly digested and burned for energy. Complex carbohydrates from beans and whole grain cereals, for instance, take longer to digest and provide a more steady delivery of fuel for your body. Your family's goal should be to eat a combination of healthy simple and complex carbohydrates from foods with the most nutrients so that you all have plenty of energy and strong, lean bodies.

FOUR EASY WAYS TO FEED YOUR FAMILY GOOD CARBS

Sugar, candy, and soft drinks all give you carbohydrates, but you probably know as well as I do that eating these foods makes you feel worse, not better. Your goal should be to eat healthy carbohydrates. For instance, an apple is packed with vitamins and fiber as well as carbs, but candy and soda are empty calories, devoid of any nutritional value. You can find healthy simple carbohydrates in fruit, dairy products, and veggies. There are healthy complex carbohydrates in beans, peas, and lentils, and whole grain breads and cereals.

Good carbs are included in all of the meals, of course, but here are my four go-to strategies for eating enough of those good carbs every day:

1. **Start your day with cereal.** I've never really been much of a junk food eater, but I've always loved cereal. I never could eat enough of it as a kid, and I'm not much different now. Cereal is a great way to jump-start your day with healthy carbohydrates, as long as you choose oatmeal or a whole grain, unsweetened cereal and have it with nonfat milk. Add blueberries, and you've got a powerfully nutritious meal.

2. **Substitute whole fruit for juice.** You love juice in the morning, and it'll certainly give you that vitamin C you're looking for. But think about substituting whole fruit for that glass of juice—you'll get the same carbs and nutrients, without the sugars.

3. **Pass on the potatoes.** Who doesn't love potatoes? But you can get a bigger dose of healthy carbs and add fiber if you swap out regular potatoes for sweet potatoes, brown rice, whole wheat pasta, or whole grain bread at lunch and dinner.

4. **Bring on the beans.** I know, I know. I sound like a broken record, bringing up beans again. But it's really tough to beat beans for a great source of healthy carbohydrates as well as protein, because your body takes a while to digest them.

7. TAKE YOUR VITAMINS—AND YOUR MINERALS, TOO

When planning a meal, most people ignore vitamins and minerals because they don't contain calories like protein, carbohydrates, and fats. No need to count the minerals and vitamins, right?

These micronutrients are absolutely necessary for ensuring the health of your family. The great thing about the *Extra Lean Family* meals is that they provide all of the micronutrients necessary to feel energetic, fend off disease, and stay in great shape.

VITAMINS	BEST SOURCES:	GOOD FOR:
Vitamin A	Dairy products, fruits, and vegetables	Promoting healthy skin, eyes, and bones
Vitamin B	Lean meats, fish, dairy, whole grains	Ensuring high protein metabolism and energy production
Vitamin C	Citrus fruits and juices	Fighting illness, building skin and tissue
Vitamin D	Dairy products and fish	Strengthening teeth and bones
Vitamin E	Green leafy vegetables, eggs, whole grains	Preventing heart disease and cancer
MINERALS		
Calcium	Dairy products, beans, leafy vegetables	Strengthening bones and muscles
Iron	Meats, fish, whole grains, dried fruit	Carrying oxygen throughout the body
Magnesium	Nuts, beans, dairy products, whole grains	Strengthening bones and muscles
Zinc	Meat, dairy products, nuts, grains	Boosting metabolism and immune system

THE SALT SHAKEDOWN

One of every family's most overlooked nutritional traps is salt. Even though adults shouldn't eat more than a teaspoon of table salt a day, the Department of Health and Human Services estimates that most Americans get nearly twice that amount. In fact, the average American's salt intake has risen 55 percent in the past decade. This is risky behavior, because a high intake of salt is linked to high blood pressure in many studies.

The American Medical Association is now urging everyone to cut back on salt in order to cut back on health issues related to high blood pressure. We need to guide our children to do the same. There has been a rise in the number of kids and teens with kidney stones, probably due to eating too much salt, and high blood pressure now affects 9 percent of overweight kids. One in every five children has high cholesterol, and the sad truth is that kids with hypertension are more likely to have heart problems as they get older.

So what can you do to put a stop to the excess amounts of salt? Here are some tips for your family:

❑ **Check food labels.** Even favorite kid foods that taste sweet, like ketchup, are loaded with salt.

❑ **Toss prepackaged rice and pasta, and cook your own.** Those little flavor packets inside the boxes of rice and pasta are usually swimming in sodium.

❑ **Choose fresh or frozen vegetables over canned.** Manufacturers use sodium to preserve canned foods and make them taste better. For instance, a can of sweet peas has 400 milligrams of salt, but a box of frozen peas has very little.

❑ **Eat potassium-rich foods.** Potassium is a powerhouse when it comes to lowering blood pressure and counterbalancing the salt in your diet. Good sources of potassium include potatoes, halibut, bananas, spinach, tomatoes, and oranges.

8. FIGHT FAT AND FEEL FIT WITH FIBER

Foods high in fiber are usually complex carbohydrates and loaded with vitamins, minerals, and other health-boosting ingredients. But fiber all by itself is a great nutrient, too, because it helps you keep body fat off, since you don't actually digest it. Instead, fiber moves through your digestive tract intact, making you feel full and curbing your appetite.

The best sources of fiber are whole grains like oatmeal and whole wheat bread, fruits, vegetables, and beans. If I need a quick, convenient snack, I'll grab an apple because it's loaded with fiber, and that will usually tide me over to my next meal. At lunch, I like to use whole grain bread for sandwiches to maximize my fiber intake. For dinner, I'll add a side of fiber-rich black beans as a great companion to a chicken breast and broccoli or pretty much any other lean protein meat and green veggie. No doubt about it, adding fiber to your diet is one of the best ways you can stay fit and *Extra Lean*.

9. UP YOUR NUTRITIONAL ARSENAL OF ANTIOXIDANTS

Simply put, an antioxidant is a micronutrient that helps prevent or slow down oxidization. Antioxidants help protect your body's cells from free radicals, those damaging substances that can cause cancer. You can easily enrich your family's diet—and boost everyone's overall health—just by adding more foods that are good sources of antioxidants, such as colorful fruits—blueberries are a great example—and vegetables, nuts and seeds, whole grains, and beans. Whenever I scramble eggs, for instance, I throw vegetables into the mix to make sure that I'm getting not just protein and vitamins, but a healthy dose of antioxidants as well. And I can't get enough blueberries. I put them on my cereal, on my oatmeal, and in my pancakes. Blueberries are also great for just snacking on between meals. Or, when I'm craving something crunchy at night, one of my favorite snacks is a handful of raw red bell pepper slices. I think of these as busy foods, because they keep my hands busy without adding extra calories, and they're busy helping my body fight disease.

10. DRINK EIGHT TO TEN GLASSES OF WATER DAILY

Probably no fuel you give your body is as important as water. Dehydration can lead to low energy, headaches, and overeating because you're compensating for being thirsty. Plus, your body relies on water to regulate your body temperature, digest your food, and keep your organs in tip-top condition.

I'm always sweating during workouts, so I drink plenty of water. Besides keeping me hydrated, water is good for my skin. I mostly drink just regular tap water and stay away from expensive vitamin waters, but once in a while, especially after a heavy workout, I'll drink a sports water.

In order to keep your body hydrated, drink eight to ten glasses per day. Encourage your children to bring water with their school lunches instead of calorie-dense, sugary juices, especially if they play sports, and keep a refillable bottle of water in the car for yourself. While other fluids will help you stay hydrated, water has them beat because your body can absorb it quickly—and without adding calories to your daily diet!

STEP 3: Know What a Healthy Plate Looks Like

In *Extra Lean*, I explained how I'd learned that one of the three key steps to eliminate unwanted fat and to keep your metabolism running high is to practice portion control. One of the simplest ways to help you and your family stay healthy, while having plenty of energy, is to know what a healthy plate looks like. The *Extra Lean Family* meal plans provide the proper amounts and balance of food that you need to control weight gain and loss. By following these meal plans for the five weeks outlined in these pages, you'll learn what a healthy plate looks like—and so will your children. That means that when a friend hands you a plate of food, or when you're served a plate in a restaurant, you will be able to tell at a glance if it has the right balance of protein, carbohydrates, and healthy fat. You'll also know right away whether the portion sizes of each type of food on your plate are the right size for you.

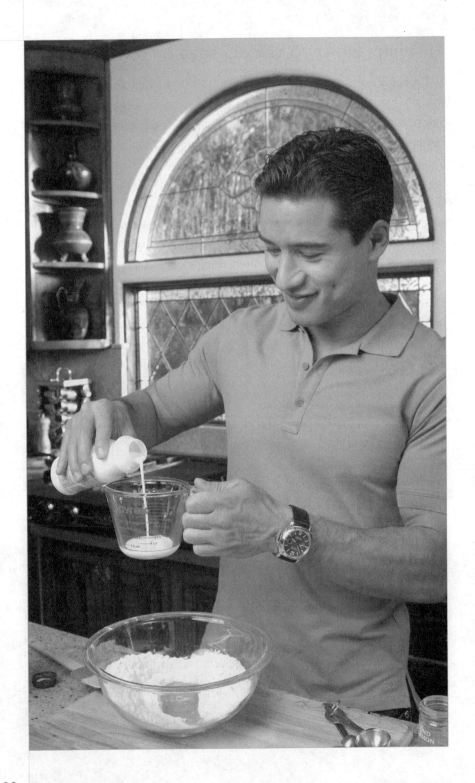

The easiest way to learn about portion size is pretty basic, as I discovered once I started really learning how to cook and paying attention to the amount of food on my plate as well as the nutritional content of that food. You just have to measure. This may sound time consuming, but trust me, measuring your food at the start of this five-week plan is key to knowing what serving sizes look like.

Adults in your family should use measuring cups to determine the right amounts of food to eat, from salad to pasta, and measuring spoons to dole out salad dressings and oils. You can also invest in a food scale to weigh meats and fish.

Eventually, you'll practice enough that you'll know by looking just how big a four ounce piece of salmon is, so that when you're at a friend's house or go out to dinner, you can monitor your portion sizes on the go. As a rough guide, you can also use the tried-and-true cheat sheet below from *Extra Lean* to help you and your family build an awareness of what portion sizes look like on a plate:

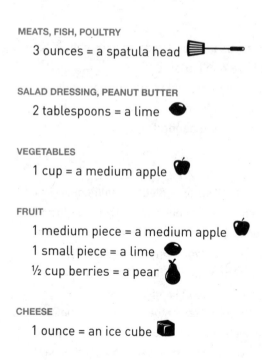

MEATS, FISH, POULTRY
  3 ounces = a spatula head

SALAD DRESSING, PEANUT BUTTER
  2 tablespoons = a lime

VEGETABLES
  1 cup = a medium apple

FRUIT
  1 medium piece = a medium apple
  1 small piece = a lime
  ½ cup berries = a pear

CHEESE
  1 ounce = an ice cube

NUTS
  ¼ cup = a lime

1 cup of popcorn or cereal = a medium apple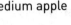

½ cup cooked rice = a lime

Your children shouldn't be counting calories. Because children are constantly growing, and adding new muscle and tissue, you certainly don't want them to diet. However, it's good for you to help them build an awareness of healthy portion sizes.

If your children are too young to understand the adult guide, help them develop their own. A great way to teach them is to use their own sticky little hands! The great thing about this system is that it works no matter how old your children are, because as their appetites grow, their hands will, too. It's also important to stick to a ten-minute rule, and ask children to wait ten minutes before taking a second helping. Then, if they really are still hungry, let them have another child-sized portion.

Here's how children of any age can measure their foods wherever they are:

A child-sized portion of meat = as long and wide as your child's palm

A child-sized portion of grains = one handful

A child-sized portion of fruits, veggies, and yogurt = one handful

A child-sized serving of cheese = a thumb

A child-sized serving of snacks = one handful

EXTRA LEAN KIDS

KIDS SHOULD NOT be on a diet. The nutritional goal for children and teens should never focus on losing weight, but on making smart changes in daily routines. For instance, you can work together as a family to get up early enough to eat a nutrition-packed breakfast—which is key to making sure your child can focus in school.

CHANGING YOUR CHILD'S behavior rather than fixating on whatever numbers are on the scale will set up your children for a lifetime of good eating habits. (That approach works well for adults, too, by the way.) Children need to be taught to make smart, nutritious food choices. They also need to pay attention to portion sizes, especially when it comes to treats like ice cream and candy, rather than seeing those foods as forbidden (which will only cause them to want them more).

ENCOURAGE YOUR CHILDREN to eat servings of the meals as they're mapped out in the book. Then, if they're still hungry, have them follow the "Ten-Minute Rule."

THE BEST THING parents can do is set a good example. Wait ten minutes after a single serving, to be sure that you're really hungry before you have a second. And you can show your children that a serving of ice cream isn't always a bad thing, but taking a spoon and a pint and finishing it off while you watch a movie on your DVR can lead to weight gain and forming bad habits. Never forget that when it comes to rules and resources for healthy eating, you're the best role model for your child.

Comprehending the metabolism and learning how to apply the principles of *Extra Lean* will ensure that you and your family speed up your metabolisms and burn off unwanted calories and fat. The ten top nutrition rules are the only resources you will ever need to fight off fat, and by recognizing what a healthy plate looks like, each member of your family will keep their metabolisms running efficiently in and out of the house. Understanding *Extra Lean Family* is to be informed about your body and metabolism and to know how to use this information to get the results you want.

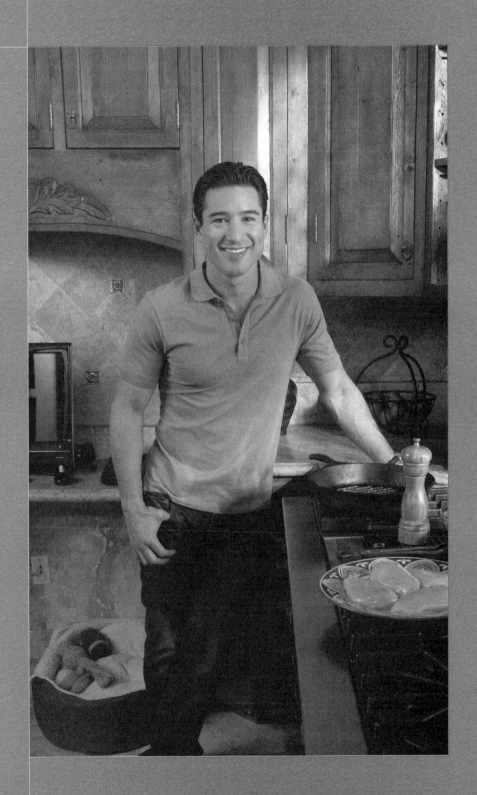

prepare for
extra lean family

Taking into account the most basic and crucial steps to control your and your family's own metabolisms, this chapter will show you how to put this knowledge to good use in preparing your family to embrace healthier eating habits and the *Extra Lean* approach to loving food.

I'll admit that this plan won't always be easy to follow. This isn't because the *Extra Lean Family* plan is complicated. The meal plan features simple, delicious, and healthy foods that can be prepared in twenty minutes or less, and provides shopping and cooking methods to make the best use of leftovers. However, preparing for *Extra Lean Family* involves your and your family's commitment to following these guidelines. That means learning to trust and support one another as you make this critical transformation to better eating habits.

This will be daunting at first. Like any family, you've already developed habits, some good, some bad. To make sure that your various trains run on time—Dad and Mom off to work, kids to school, plus fitting in social events, sports, and extracurricular activities—there's very little time left in the day to stop, refocus, and figure out what's working right for your family and what could use a little more attention.

The best place to start is with a nutrition intervention plan, an easy three-step guide that will help you and your family set goals for healthier living and reach them. First, you and your family will reevaluate the foods that you eat now by keeping a food journal—necessary for making this much-needed transition! This chapter will provide tangible and specific tips on how to make the most of this simple yet highly effective tool. Second, you'll learn how to give your kitchen a complete makeover so that you can toss out bad habits and prepare to adopt the good habits that the meal plan naturally instills. Third, I'll show you how to navigate through the grocery store so that you stay focused on your goals while shopping for the items in the meal plan and beyond.

STEP 1: Reevaluate the Foods You Eat

To optimize your metabolism, you'll need to examine your own eating habits and reevaluate the foods you eat. This first step is key to successfully following the five-week meal plan as you begin committing yourself and your family to a healthier lifestyle.

When I hit my mid-twenties, I woke up one day and saw that I looked a little huskier on TV. I was still working out a lot, but I was also eating the same foods that I'd always eaten as a teenager. I didn't feel like my activity level had gone down any, but it was clear that my metabolism was starting to change. I couldn't just keep eating the same foods, in the same amounts, that I'd been eating my whole life.

That was when I had to admit that no fitness regimen in the world could possibly help me stay healthy and lean. I needed to change my eating habits. I started deliberately making a note of everything I ate, every time I ate, and that helped me develop a new awareness of what I was putting into my body.

You and your family can take notes, too, as part of setting up and successfully meeting your goals. Food journals are a great way to document what your habits are now and to start looking more objectively at the foods you eat, when you eat them, and even why you've gotten into the habit of eating particular foods. After a while, you'll build up your internal awareness of portion sizes and what nutrients you're currently putting on your plate—and in your body—at every meal. That awareness will go a long way in getting your family's discussion about healthy eating started.

Every family is different, and every family member is unique. But here are key strategies for keeping a food journal that will help you and your family prepare yourselves for *Extra Lean* living:

1. Start your family food journal the week before you begin cooking the recipes in this book. This will help each person in your family spot weaknesses and strengths in the food choices your family makes now.

2. Choose five rules from the Top Ten Nutrition Rules for Boosting Your Metabolism in Chapter 1 and make these your goals to accomplish each day. Rotate the rules for each day of the week so that you can make use of all ten.

3. Then, as you and your family write down what each of you ate at the end of the day, either in a common notebook or on the family computer, evaluate how your actual actions matched up to the ten nutrition rules you set as your goals. This will help you determine what foods and habits you need to eliminate to increase your metabolism and what you are already doing that benefits your body and metabolism. Because the five-week *Extra Lean Family* meal plan incorporates these nutrition rules into every meal, your family will more likely recognize the healthful benefits of cooking the recipes after keeping a journal, and everyone will be more likely to commit to the plan.

Remember, each person's goals will be different. You may want to lose twenty pounds, and reading the family food journal might help you see that you always reach for carbohydrates when you're stressed about work, or that you've been loading up your salads with Ranch dressing when you could be using just a little oil and vinegar. Meanwhile, your high school soccer player is keen on gaining muscle, and reading the journal might help him see that he's coming up short on protein, so he can't possibly build up the muscles he needs. Or maybe your daughter is gorging on sweets instead of snacks packed with nutrition between school and swim practice.

As you get into the *Extra Lean Family* plan and start using the recipes, keep your journal up for another week or two—or for as long as you think it's useful. Keeping your journal will help each of you be accountable, and it won't take long before each person starts self-correcting and making healthier choices even when they're not at home.

If you want to lose weight, for instance, keeping a journal of all of your daily meals will let you know how close you're coming to your ideal daily calorie count. If you go down a dress size, you can look at your journal and know without a doubt that your food choices are working to help you accomplish your goals.

Midway through the *Extra Lean Family* plan, your family can have fun reading your food journal entries from the very beginning. I'm betting that you'll see a big change in your family's awareness and food choices. Keeping a food journal will help prepare everyone in your family to think, live, and eat as an *Extra Lean Family*.

EXTRA LEAN FACT

PEOPLE WHO KEEP food journals lose twice as much weight as those who don't. That's because keeping a food journal allows you to monitor the types of foods you eat at certain times. It's easy to pinpoint the problem and solution when you know which types of foods contribute to weight gain and which types boost your metabolism. A food journal is a great tool for truly understanding your food habits, which is the key to unraveling your body's metabolism.

STEP 2: Give Your Kitchen an *Extra Lean Family* Makeover

We all have our go-to foods. These are the foods that we always keep on hand so that we can grab a snack we like when we have to rush out the door to meet a friend, or the ingredients we always use to cook a quick dinner if company decides to show up. For instance, I always have everything I need to make my favorite whole wheat penne pasta with some grilled, chopped up chicken sausages, a little balsamic vinegar, olive oil, and a dash of lime juice.

I know from my own experience of learning to enjoy different foods with a lot more awareness of what kind of fuel I'm putting into my body that it's easier to stick to your goals if you turn your kitchen into a healthy place to be. This is where meals are created, and if you don't provide the right building blocks of nutritious ingredients, it's all too tempting to order takeout or fall back on what's familiar. Takeout and packaged foods give us a shortcut, but as you've already seen, they're also loaded with sugar, unhealthy saturated fats, and salt. Now that you've evaluated the types of foods you should curb and the types of foods you should integrate into your everyday diet, you're ready to give your kitchen a healthy makeover. The good news is that this is a lot less expensive than knocking down walls and changing the paint. The bad news is that it can be a little complicated. But don't worry. I'm going to walk you through the process of creating your very own *Extra Lean* kitchen.

This part will require a little work, but it's definitely worth the effort: Take every single thing out of your cupboard and pantry, shelf by shelf, drawer by drawer. What do you see? Takeout containers? Soda bottles? Packaged foods? Sugary cereals? Are the drawers and shelves packed with fruits and vegetables, or not so much? What about your freezer? Do you have anything in there you could pull out for a healthy dinner? Or are the shelves crammed with ice cream and TV dinners?

The main goal here should be to help assess your starting point. Some of these foods will have to go, and it's better to just drop them into the trash can or compost bin right now than to go on one last binge to empty your fridge. Read the food labels on everything you're uncertain about, and that will help make up your mind about whether a certain box or can has to go.

Here are my top five kitchen makeover rules:

1. **Trash the trans fats.** There are so many sources of these bad fats in most kitchens that, even if you took no other step in making over your kitchen besides this one, your family would already be healthier. Here are some examples of common foods that are typically loaded with trans fats: Packaged foods like cake mixes; ramen noodles and those instant soup cups your kids love; margarine; many frozen pizzas, pies, and chicken nuggets; doughnuts and commercially baked products; crackers and potato chips; many breakfast cereals.

2. **Consider your condiments.** Mayonnaise can pack in a lot of calories and saturated fat if consumed in large amounts, so the next time you go shopping, grab the smallest jar to avoid overuse. If you are a huge fan of chicken salad or tuna salad, replace half of the mayo with nonfat yogurt, and you'll still get that creamy texture with less fat. If you want to take mayo out of your diet completely, you can spread hummus or avocado in your sandwiches to give them some texture and taste. Soy sauce and teriyaki sauce are loaded with sodium. For the former, switch to low sodium and try making the latter on your own. Most ketchups are loaded with sugar and artificial ingredients. Look for an organic version with more natural ingredients. Again, read the food labels to decide whether or not a certain condiment deserves a place in your healthy kitchen.

3. **Switch to healthier cooking oils.** To achieve your best health, you need to start cooking with the least amount of trans fat and saturated fat possible, and add in omega-3s and monounsaturated fats. You should cook mostly with canola oil, which contains the lowest amount of saturated fat and is loaded with omega-3 fatty acids, or with olive oil, which has more monounsaturated fat than any other oil. Olive oil also tastes great.

I've become an even bigger fan of olive oil since meeting Gia Francesca's mom, who's such a fantastic cook and loves to prepare Italian dishes.

4. **Make easy substitutions.** You don't want your family to feel deprived. As soon as you dejunk your pantry and refrigerator, make it over with some easy, tasty, healthy substitutions like these: Low fat, low sugar, whole grain breakfast cereals and granola bars instead of Pop Tarts and sugary cereal bars; mustard for mayonnaise; low-salt mixed nuts and reduced-fat whole grain crackers for potato chips; whole grain pretzels for regular pretzels.

5. **Out with the bad, in with the good.** Once you get to the meal plans, you'll find complete shopping lists to help you plan and prepare each week's healthy meals without effort. Besides that, though, you'll want to do what I do and always have a few healthy cooking basics on hand that you'll use over and over again. Before each trip to the store, I take a quick survey of my kitchen to make sure that I have these items in stock, because I know I'll need them:

White Whole Wheat Flour: This flour looks and tastes like white flour, so your kids won't know the difference. But it has three times as much fiber. Substitute it in any recipe!

Low Sodium Chicken Broth: Chicken broth is useful for so many things, so you'll want to have it on hand. Choosing a brand that has the least amount sodium will help drastically reduce the unhealthy salt in your family's diet.

Spices: Even the most boring meals come alive with no-calorie spices. Make sure you have cumin, coriander, cinnamon, and turmeric.

Oils: The healthiest oils for cooking and salad dressings are extra-virgin olive oil and canola oil. Buy the plain kind, not the flavored, to save money. You can spice it up yourself.

Low Sodium Soy Sauce: A stir-fry dinner is quick to make, as you'll see in my menu plan. But most soy sauces are unhealthy because they're so high in sodium. Look for a low sodium brand.

Garlic & Onions: Flavor is what I'm always after, and nothing adds it like garlic and onion. Plus, they're calorie-free!

Instant Brown Rice: Many of my recipes call for brown rice. Instant brown rice has the same amount of fiber and whole grains as the slow version.

Canned Beans: Nothing beats beans if you're adding protein and iron to any meal. Just be sure to buy the low-salt ones and rinse them thoroughly before use.

Healthy Pasta: Many kids won't eat whole wheat or spinach pasta, but there are many brands made with oats, flax seed, and lentils that will taste about the same but be much better for them.

Pasta Sauce: You'll probably want to make your own to save money and be sure it's as healthy as possible. However, if you're in a pinch for time, have a jar of organic tomato sauce on hand that's low in salt and added sugar.

Canned Tomatoes: Believe it or not, canned tomatoes actually have more of the antioxidant lycopene than fresh. Keep canned tomatoes on hand for chili and tacos, or to add to almost any pasta or vegetable for flavor.

Cereal and Cereal Bars: Always check the food labels on cereals, because so many are high in sugar. Try to buy only whole grain cereals with fewer than eight grams of sugar per serving.

Dried Fruit: Cherries, raisins, and other dried fruits can be rich in antioxidants. If your kids don't like the soft, leathery dried fruits, check out the crunchy kind.

Granola Bars: You don't want sugar to be the first ingredient on the label of your granola bar—then you might as well be eating cookies. You also don't want to buy granola bars that are high in trans fat. I usually choose a granola bar that's a little higher in calories with nuts and dried fruits, instead of those chewy chocolate-chip ones, because I want the extra nutrients.

Fresh and Frozen Fruit: I can't think of any time when it's a bad idea to have fruit as a snack or to add extra nutrition to your salad. I always have fresh fruit out on the counter to tempt me to grab an apple or a banana for a snack instead of something that won't fuel my body as efficiently. I like to keep frozen mixed fruit in the freezer, too, because I'm always up for a fruit smoothie.

Frozen Fish: I try to always buy my fish the same day I'm going to eat it. But I like to eat fish a couple of times a week, and you never know when company is going to stop by, or when bad weather or a hectic schedule might keep you from making it to the store like you'd planned. It's great to have fish fillets in the freezer that you can pull out in a hurry, since they're so quick to thaw and cook, and still packed with healthy omega-3 fatty acids.

Juices: I try to keep only natural juices on hand. Look for real, unsweetened fruit juice as the main ingredient, and get as close to 100 percent as you can—then dilute it with water when you drink it.

Natural Peanut Butter: Natural peanut butter may take some getting used to, because it's not as sweet as the other brands, but it's definitely worth it. Nothing picks a kid up like a PB&J or peanut butter on crackers after school with a glass of milk.

Popcorn: This is a whole grain treat! Use low-salt brands.

You'll also want to make sure that you have healthy herbs ready at hand. The *Extra Lean Family* recipes are low in fat and calories, but high on flavor. That's because I always make sure to add herbs and spices for excitement. There's another reason, too: a lot of the herbs I rely on pack an added nutritional punch. Here's a list of my absolute favorite healthy herbs:

- ❑ **Basil:** Probably no herb packs as many antioxidants as basil. Basil is rich in vitamins A, C, and K, as well as calcium, iron, and potassium. You can make pesto to spoon over chicken breasts or stir into pasta. Toss two teaspoons of basil onto your pizza to get 5 percent of your daily requirement of magnesium—that's a mighty mineral that works to restore normal muscle and nerve function. Or, if your kids hate little green specks in their meals, grind up basil until it is super fine, then add it to sauces and soups.
- ❑ **Cilantro:** I grew up eating my mom's homemade Mexican food, so you can bet that I had a lot of cilantro in my meals as a child. Mom loved to stir this green herb into salsa to top our tacos and so do I. Cilantro is also great in soups and salads. It will help aid your family's digestion, and studies show that this plant accelerates the removal of excess toxic metals from the body.
- ❑ **Dill:** I love dill in just about anything, but especially for flavoring fish. If you add dill to your tuna salad or to your salmon, you're helping your family maintain healthy cholesterol levels. Dill also can soothe digestion.
- ❑ **Parsley:** I love dressing up a plate with parsley—it adds great color and texture, and the taste of this leafy herb can really bump up the flavor of sauces and salads. Plus, parsley packs a lot of vitamin K—important for healthy blood clotting—and vitamins C and A.
- ❑ **Rosemary:** Sprinkle rosemary on turkey or chicken breasts to boost the flavor—and to help cut your family's cancer risk. Rosemary has special antioxidants that can help combat the carcinogens potentially created by grilling or broiling meat at temperatures above 400 degrees.
- ❑ **Thyme:** Besides adding color and zest to sauces and meats, thyme sprinkled into a salad dressing or added to your favorite soups and stews can help you ramp up your intake of daily iron.

A lot of people add it to tea as well, especially to ease coughs and sore throats.

STEP 3: Shop Lean and Wisely

By knowing what to keep in and what to throw out of your kitchen, you'll make grocery shopping much easier to tackle. You've probably had the same experience I've had, where you've had unexpected company over the weekend, you stop at the store to buy a dozen eggs because you've run out sooner than you'd planned, and suddenly everything looks good to you. Maybe you're hungry because it's just after work, or the children are crabby and begging for everything they see, and pretty soon you have a cart full of food you don't need.

Everyone wants to save money on their grocery bills, and the great thing about the plan is that you are buying only what you need and what's good for you. First of all, you'll find complete shopping lists included right here in this book for every single meal. Secondly, if you're keen on saving money on food, I've given you some great ways to use leftovers and make entirely new meals, so that you can buy food in bigger quantities and save a little money there.

Here are some things that have worked for me:

>> It's best to shop only when you have a list for the week's recipes—and only after you've checked your kitchen to see what you already have on hand in the house. That list will save you from being lured by items that are on sale—but that you don't use or need.

>> If you're making your own list, organize your list by food category. Or, you can list foods in the same order as your store's aisle layout. That will help you avoid temptation and get in and out of the store faster.

>> Never shop when you're hungry!

>> Try a few different stores in your neighborhood and keep a price log in a small notebook, recording the best prices of your favorite items when you shop at each store. After doing this, you'll

know which store has the best bargains on the foods your family eats most often.

>> Use a smaller cart or even a basket if you can. Having more room in your cart will tempt you to fill it.

>> Invest in some clear see-through storage containers for leftovers, so that you always know what's in the refrigerator and freezer. You'll waste less food that way.

THE PRACTICAL GUIDE TO SHOPPING ORGANIC:
WHEN IS IT NECESSARY, AND WHEN IS IT JUST A SPLURGE?

I can't remember when most grocery stores started having health food aisles and touting "organic" foods, but it's been long enough that many Americans—at least two-thirds—buy some organic produce and meat every time they go to the grocery store. These products are almost always more costly than foods that aren't organic—sometimes even double the price.

Food that meets government standards for "organic" includes food that hasn't been genetically modified or irradiated. In addition, organic meat is from animals that have had access to the outdoors; haven't been fed feed made from animal by-products or treated with antibiotics or growth hormones; and have eaten only organic feed for at least a year. Organic produce hasn't been exposed to pesticides made from synthetic chemicals.

To earn that organic label, a food must be made of at least 95 percent organic ingredients. Foods can also be "made with organic ingredients" if 70 percent of the ingredients are organic. "Natural" and even "all natural" foods are not necessarily organic; there is no official government standard for these terms.

For my family, I do try to buy some organic foods, but I don't go crazy. I consider it a good idea to spend extra money for organic baby food, apples, berries, dairy products, eggs, imported grapes, and meat. If money isn't tight, go ahead and buy other organic produce, too. Studies have shown that it's really tough to wash chemicals off of produce no matter how many times you rinse it; if you can't buy organic produce, then peel it. Because there aren't really any government standards for organic seafood, I don't waste money on that.

Here's my breakdown on what's necessary, and what's a splurge, when it comes to buying organic food:

NECESSARY
Apples
Baby food
Berries
Grapes
Dairy
Eggs
Meat
Spinach

A SPLURGE, BUT GOOD TO GO ORGANIC, IF POSSIBLE, ON:
Avocados
Broccoli
Corn
Kiwi
Mangoes
Oils
Pasta
Dried fruit

A WASTE OF MONEY
Seafood
Bananas

>> Avoid temptation. Don't go down any grocery aisle unless there's something on your list that's down that aisle.
>> Buy steaks in the winter when nobody's got their backyard grills up and running, because they're cheaper then. The same goes

for roasts: hardly anyone roasts meat in the summer, so that meat is cheaper in the summer months.

>> Whenever the meats that you use a lot do go on sale, buy a lot of it and bring it home, then rewrap it into one-pound packages (or whatever size your family needs for most meals) and freeze them for future use.

>> Buying a whole chicken is cheaper than buying chicken already cut into pieces. You can cook a whole chicken and then debone it to get enough meat for three family meals: a casserole, a soup, and fajitas.

>> Whenever you see boneless, skinless chicken breast on sale, buy it and store it in heavy-duty freezer bags in the amounts your family needs, then freeze it. Frozen chicken can last for months and is always a great thing to have on hand for a quick meal.

>> Having said all of the above about buying meat in quantity when it's on sale, it's also key to remember that bigger isn't necessarily better. Be careful of "value size" packages. Always read the prices on items to see if it's really a better deal, and make sure you'll use the item in the amount you'll buy.

>> Frozen vegetables are actually just as nutritious as fresh, because frozen vegetables are flash-frozen. Plus, frozen veggies tend to be cheaper.

>> If you have a small family, buy lettuce at a salad bar so that you can buy it in smaller amounts and won't waste half a head of uneaten lettuce.

>> If your kids love oatmeal, but you don't really have time to fix it in the morning, make a huge pot on Sunday morning, then store the oatmeal in a large sealed container and microwave it as you need it.

>> If you know that certain nonfood items, like wrapping paper or greeting cards, can be purchased for less money somewhere else, don't buy them at the grocery store. Just shop for the foods you need and get out.

>> Mix your own granola.

>> Don't be loyal to any single brand. Buy store brands or brands on sale.

>> If you always buy the same magazines at the grocery store, stop right now and subscribe for a year.

>> If something is on sale and says "6 for $10," but you need only one or two of those items, you can almost always still buy them at the sale price. You don't need to buy six.

>> Before you proceed to the checkout counter, survey the items in your cart. Is there anything there that wasn't on your list? Do you really need it? If not, take it out and put it back!

>> Finally, once you're in the checkout line, don't stoop to impulse purchases. You can buy batteries or whatever else they have by the cash register more cheaply somewhere else.

THE LOWDOWN
ON FOOD LABELS

It's already a lot of work to get to the grocery store, then come home and put things away. Reading food labels? Who has the time?

We all do, and we all should. I can't think of a better way to promote healthy eating for your family than actually stepping up and reading the labels on the food you eat to find out what's really going on your family's table—or in their lunch bags and bedtime snacks. If your children are old enough, give them practice reading the labels and discuss what ingredients are actually in their favorite foods. That way, you can help them build an awareness of how important it is to understand our foods and make healthy choices for themselves.

Food labels give you all kinds of useful information. Every package of food you buy—whether it's a bag, a box, or a can—has information about serving sizes; calories; the amount of fat, protein, carbohydrates, and vitamins in that food; and an ingredients list. Basically, the top part of a food label typically contains information about serving size, calories, and nutrient information. The bottom part of every food label should give you the daily vitamin and mineral values for 2,000–2,500 calorie diets.

Sounds good, right? Well, yes, it is great to be informed, but you also need to read between the lines on food labels. For instance, a label that claims a food has "0 grams trans fat"—remember, those are the bad fats that you don't want to give your family—doesn't mean that food is necessarily free of other bad fats, or that the food necessarily has healthy polyunsaturated fat. Some foods really are loaded with bad saturated fats, and you need to read the label carefully to know that before you buy that particular food.

Food labels that scream "all natural!" sound good, but you should still look at the ingredients list. Even products with manufactured high fructose corn syrup—another thing you want to steer away from for the sake of your family's health—are allowed to make this "all natural" claim by the government.

Another tricky label is the one that may say "made with 100 percent fruit." No matter what that food is, it's not as healthy for your family as actual fruit. After all, the product might be made with 100 percent fruit, but if the fruit makes up only 2 percent of the product, that's really not much nutrition. You'd do better handing everyone in your family an actual apple.

You can check out the U.S. Food and Drug Administration's detailed guide to reading food labels at their Web site, http://www.fda.gov/Food/Labeling-Nutrition/ConsumerInformation/ucm078889.htm. In general, though, when you're reading food labels, you want to make sure to look up any ingredient name you're unfamiliar with, and follow this guide:

- Avoid any foods that are processed with a lot of sodium, like frozen dinners and packaged snacks.
- Avoid foods with processed sweeteners and added sugars. There are lots of names for added sugars, like evaporated cane juice or high fructose corn syrup.
- Choose foods that are low in saturated fat and free of trans fats; look carefully at the label to make sure the food you buy has healthy mono and polyunsaturated fats.
- Choose foods that have at least 3 grams of fiber per serving if possible.
- Choose foods without trans fats—these are often listed as "partially hydrogenated oils" on the ingredients list.

Keeping a food journal with your family will help each of you reevaluate what you eat and assess how you can boost your metabolism. Once you've prepared your bodies and minds, and you've gotten your kitchen ready, too, eliminate unhealthy processed and fatty foods and substitute nutritious ones so that any time you cook a meal or make a snack, you'll have all the ingredients and flavor boosters that will help you curb the fat and boost your metabolism. By learning some valuable shopping tips to keep focused and on track and save time and money, you'll have invaluable resources that will prevent you from falling off the five week plan and beyond.

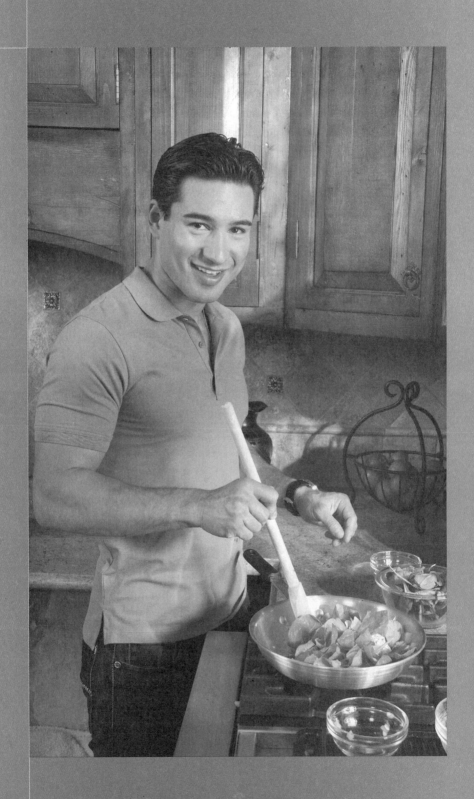

maintain
extra lean family

IT'S EASY TO let your busy routine and everyday life interrupt your goals. It's not that most people refuse to make the healthy transition, but rather that time and commitment on top of an already hectic schedule makes the effort of eating better as a family seem an impossible challenge. I know firsthand what this feels like. I'm constantly darting from one set to another, and when I'm not at the office, I'm traveling. Now that I'm also juggling the role of fatherhood, I've definitely had to rethink my whole approach to eating since I'm not only responsible for my own health but for my family's as well.

In this chapter, you'll learn tangible and practical ways to maintain your focus while you change your family's approach to food through preparing and cooking the recipes. From my own experience trying to maintain and instill good eating habits in my family, I've discovered that to constantly achieve lean and healthy results, everyone in the household has to 1) understand why every meal matters, 2) plan ahead, and 3) prepare and eat meals as a family.

Understanding why every meal matters has helped me make better choices when it comes to food. In my line of work, there are times during the year when I'm hardly at home and I've had to figure out a way to eat well when I'm on set, on the road, or even at a restaurant. In this section, I break down why and how each meal contributes to a high metabolism and explain how you can make the most of balancing your foods and nutrients for each meal.

Planning ahead is pretty much an imperative for all the important things in life, and food is no exception. If you get a head start at the beginning of the week, you're more likely to follow through with the meal plan and succeed in your efforts toward healthy eating. The beauty of the meal plan is that it's designed specifically for busy households and you'll learn time-saving strategies for feeding your hungry brood while maintaining your family's short- and long-term health goals.

Preparing and eating meals with your family is the best way you can show your children how to adopt a healthy view of food. Involving them in the preparation process will make them appreciate a variety of good food, and with the cooking tips listed in this section, you and your family will learn invaluable methods to cook quick, healthy, and delicious meals for life.

STEP 1: Understand Why Every Meal Matters

Most people have good intentions when it comes to eating habits. We don't want to eat fatty, processed foods, but we're so often in a rush that we sometimes skip a meal altogether.

The problem with skipping meals is that you're most likely to head for your favorite fast food spot or buy prepackaged meals from the grocery store if you're strapped for time. Both of these options are more unhealthy than the meals and snacks you prepare yourself, because instant dinners and fast foods are typically high in calories, loaded with unwanted fats and carbs, high in salt and those "bad" trans fats, and low on nutrition.

With the *Extra Lean Family* meal plan, you can have the best of both worlds: health and convenience. You can prepare every meal in this book in twenty minutes or fewer. In each week's meal plan, I'll also show you how to jump-start your meal preparation on Sunday to save time.

In addition, because I enjoyed eating with my family while I was growing up, and I know how important it is for all children to benefit from this family ritual, I've made a point of featuring meals that every family member will enjoy. I've even included desserts that are delicious but won't derail your family's goals to be leaner and healthier.

You may still be secretly thinking that you can skip a few meals here and there, especially if your goal is to lose weight. Let's examine the importance of each meal here and see if I can change your mind.

BREAKFAST: Did you know that studies show that people who skip breakfast tend to be more overweight than those who eat breakfast every morning? No matter how rushed your family routine is in the morning, make sure to eat a breakfast that contains good carbs, protein, and healthy fat, whether that means spending fifteen minutes poaching an egg and putting it on a slice of wheat toast or five minutes blending a smoothie that your teenager can drink in the car on the way to school.

Why does breakfast matter so much? Think of it as setting your metabolism up for the day. Your body is in a fasting state because you've been asleep for eight hours or so. When you fast, your metabolism slows down to conserve energy. And, as I've touched on before, the slower your metabolism, the fewer calories and fat you're going to burn at rest. Feeding your body first thing in the morning will jump-start your body's furnace and get your metabolism going as efficiently as possible.

If you get the right nutrients into your body from the start, you've already got a great store of energy that you can draw on throughout the morning. You'll work better and your children will learn better in school, because food is fuel for the brain as well as for the body.

As for what type of food is best at breakfast, eggs are a good call. Eggs contain both protein and healthy fats that provide energy. You'll see a lot of eggs worked into the meal plan—scrambled with vegetables and turkey, or just poached. The meals deliver complex carbohydrates in all the breakfast recipes, too, because those carbohydrates provide long-lasting physical and mental energy. You also need the vitamins and minerals from fruit. In the breakfast recipes, you'll see carb-enriched, kid-friendly meals like French toast, whole grain cereal with fruit, oatmeal and orange juice, and a banana with a whole wheat English muffin, among others.

LUNCH: Breakfast may be your most important meal of the day, but as any school kid knows, it's important not to shortchange lunch. Lunch is the most pivotal meal because the second half of your family's busy work or school day depends on what you all eat for your midday meal. If you skip lunch, or if you have a lunch high on calories but low on nutrition, you're apt to feel sluggish or crave a nap. If you eat a nutritious lunch, on the other hand, you'll feel alert and have higher energy.

Finding that nutrition at lunchtime can be tough if you're out of the house, simply because there are so many unhealthy temptations. Your kids will most likely be eating in the school cafeteria, where the choices may be unappealing, or they'll be goofing off with friends and won't have time to eat. Coworkers are apt to invite you to dine out at restaurants where menus are loaded with fried foods. Or, if you're busy and can't leave the office, you may resort to vending machine options—also high in calories and low on nutrients. Your kids will haunt the vending machines at school, too, in search of calories to fill their empty stomachs if they didn't like what was on that lunch tray.

Packing lunch is the surest way to get the best nutrition. In the lunch menus, you'll see some great choices that are designed to offer the right portion sizes and all of the wholesome nutrients everybody needs to get through the day, like a turkey and avocado pita, a chef's salad, or even a surprisingly healthy, energy-packed peanut butter and jam sandwich on wheat bread.

SNACKS: I've talked about the misconceptions people have had about snacking between meals, and how eating several small meals throughout the day is the best way to stay lean and healthy. Snacking is absolutely necessary if you're going to keep your metabolism going and burn off calories in the most efficient way possible. I don't think of snacks as being much different from regular meals, truthfully, except that they're smaller. Just think of your snacks as a quick way to recharge your battery to keep your energy level and your metabolism revving, and you're on the right track.

The pitfall here is that so many foods that we consider snacks are sugary goodies that are heavy on carbs but low on other nutrients, especially the snacks that kids love and that are so easy to buy and toss into their backpacks because those processed snacks are neatly packaged. Those packaged snacks are especially deadly, because they're heavily processed and contain unhealthy trans fats and high levels of salt. If you don't pack snacks for you or your child during the day, you're apt to pull out money for the vending machine or stop at the corner store, and the last time I looked, those places didn't offer a lot of fruit and vegetables. That kind of poor planning leads to both kids and parents making bad food decisions.

If you make snacks a priority rather than an afterthought, you're more likely to have healthy choices available. I've listed lots of great snack options in this menu plan, but when in doubt, choose fruit, vegetables, and nuts to give you sustained energy.

DINNER: When it comes to family bonding time, few rituals top the family dinner for importance to overall health. A nutritious meal at the end of the day is also a strong finish to a day that started right with a good breakfast and gained momentum in the afternoon with a great lunch. This is the last substantial meal you should eat, too, so it's important to make it count.

Dinner can be tricky. Whereas there are consistent foods people eat at breakfast or lunch, like eggs and cereal, that they may not even consider having later in the day, all bets are off for dinner. Plus, the commitment to controlling your portion sizes may waver, especially if you feel like you've been "good" for the rest of the day. People are prone to overeat at dinner, and the best way to avoid that is to follow the meal plan and avoid cooking too much food. The meal plans are designed to feed four people. Don't go overboard and cook a meal that feeds eight if there are only four people in your family unless you're planning to turn the leftovers into another meal.

The dinner recipes here will show you just how much to make, and there are lots of fantastic family favorites like burgers, pork chops, and enchiladas that your family can enjoy, absolutely guilt free, because they're in reasonable portion sizes and made with the healthiest ingredients possible.

STEP 2: Plan Your Week

When are you most likely to reach for the wrong snack or feel most tempted to turn into that familiar fast food drive-through lane? By now, you know the answer as well as I do: It usually happens when you're short on time.

Planning ahead every week to determine what you'll eat for that week is the best way to stop feeling overwhelmed—and to prevent anything from derailing you from eating *Extra Lean*.

You've already started planning your week with your kitchen make-over. Now that you have healthy foods in your kitchen, you're going to double-check your fridge and shelves to see exactly what's there, and then make a list before you go to the store. You'll want to write down exactly what you need so that you won't waste money on foods that are going to spoil, and you won't be trying to cook a meal without having the necessary ingredients on hand.

Among the best features of this book are the weekly shopping lists that I've put together for you, so that you don't have to go through every meal at the beginning of the week and decide what to buy. Simply photo-copy the page and bring the list with you.

With my busy schedule, I don't have two hours to spend shopping for food, and I'm sure you don't, either. I want to get in and out of the store in less than an hour with everything I need for the week, so that I don't have to go back to the store midweek for things I've forgotten. That's why I've taken the time not only to make lists for you, but to break them down into different food categories, from dairy to produce, so that you can navigate the grocery store aisles as efficiently as possible.

In terms of planning your week, also featured in the meal plans are Sunday Prep Days to help you stay ahead of your food schedule and to maximize use of your groceries for the week. Tips include purchasing a rotisserie chicken and shredding the meat for enchiladas and wraps, making brown rice to last for the whole week, and using leftover chicken to create homemade stock. Devoting just a couple of hours on Sunday to prep foods will save you some valuable time during the week and ensure that you stay on track with the plan.

Finally, one of my favorite features of the meal plan is the Double Duty option in each week. Not everyone has the same preferences for food, so I made it a point to make the meals as intriguing as possible. The Double Duty options are key to keeping your family satisfied and interested in the foods because it offers you different variations of meals that use the same main ingredients. This way, you can please all the different eaters in the family while still using the same items on the shopping list for that particular week. The Double Duty option is just another important method of introducing variety and keeping everyone happy and satisfied.

STEP 3: Prepare and Eat Meals as a Family

Your chances of succeeding with the *Extra Lean Family* plan will ramp right up if you all continue working together to achieve your goals. Everyone should have a say in the family's nutrition and fitness plan, your family should eat and exercise together as often as possible, and—perhaps most importantly—everyone should pitch in when it comes to meal preparation. All children love to feel like they're contributing to the family. In addition, kids are much more likely to try a wider variety of foods if they're involved in choosing and preparing them. These children are also more likely to maintain healthier adult diets.

The more you can engage your children in the process of planning meals, the more they'll learn about proper eating habits and the more they'll "own" the foods they eat. They'll take pride and joy in fixing food with you as a family. If you can take them to a local farm to pick produce, or even to a farmers' market to meet the people who grow the foods you're going to put on the table together, they'll become much more invested in the *Extra Lean Family* plan and in healthy eating overall.

If you grew up like I did, your parents and grandparents probably didn't spare the butter, oil, or margarine when they were cooking. Why would they, right? They'd tell you that butter and oil gave your food great flavor and kept it from sticking to the pans.

The problem is, cooking in lots of butter and oil makes your food fattier, and can turn even the healthiest vegetables into terrible food choices if you prepare them that way. As you follow the five-week meal plan, you'll discover that you don't have to eat dry, skinless, bland foods to eat *Extra Lean*. I use a lot of cooking techniques that actually help seal in flavor without sacrificing nutrition or adding unnecessary, unhealthy fats. My methods are fast, too! Here are my personal favorites:

Sautéing: I love to sauté food because it's so quick. Use a nonstick skillet and a small amount of canola or olive oil; you can also combine the oil with a little chicken broth. If the food starts sticking, add a little water or broth. Be sure to heat the oil in the pan before you start cooking to avoid having the food absorb the oil. You can test to see if the pan is hot enough by tossing a few drops of water in with your fingertips. If the water sizzles, your pan is ready!

Oven-Frying: This is a great cooking technique because you can cook so many foods that your family loves in a much healthier way. All of those foods that we've grown up eating as deep fried, or even pan-fried, like breaded chicken and batter-dipped veggies, can be oven-fried to keep them *Extra Lean*. For breaded foods, just coat the food with egg whites (eliminating the yolk cuts down on cholesterol and fat), then slide it through your breading. Bake it on a nonstick pan at a high heat—450 degrees—until crisp.

Steaming: If you need to cook fish, vegetables, or other delicate foods, you can use moist heat and save on calories and fat. If you don't have a steamer basket, I highly recommend that you go to your local department store or kitchen store and buy one. To steam food, just bring an inch of water to a rapid boil in a saucepan, place the food in the steamer basket, and put the steamer basket into the pan. (The food shouldn't touch the water.) Cover the pan, lower the heat, and steam the food until it's cooked. The other thing I like to do is steam foods in the oven. You can do this by wrapping chicken or fish in foil and baking at 400 degrees until the food is cooked. You can add citrus juice, spices, veggies, or whatever else you like to the packets for extra flavor.

Poaching: I love to poach eggs and fish. I poach chicken sometimes, too, that I'll later shred and use in dishes or sandwiches. Poached food is cooked like steamed food, only forget the steamer basket and put the food right into the water. You can season the water, too, with spices, lemon juice, or orange juice—whatever flavor you like, just toss some into the water.

Roasting: If you roast food, you can still get great flavors but you don't have to use all of that oil or butter. For instance, if you want to make vegetables, you can do them right in the oven. Just put the veggies in a single layer in a baking dish, add seasonings and a small amount of olive oil, and cook them on the lowest shelf of your oven at 500 degrees until they're just as crispy as you like them. Most vegetables take twenty to thirty minutes. Kids will gobble up roasted veggies like they're French fries!

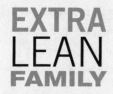

EXTRA LEAN FAMILY *tip*

YOU CAN TURN pretty much any *Extra Lean* food into an extra exciting, high flavor fiesta. Just add what I call "flavor boosters" when you cook. These flavor boosters make the recipes in my book extra nutritious and colorful—without adding unnecessary calories or unhealthy fats. If you want to play around with flavor boosters in your own recipes, here's a great list of my favorites:

CITRUS JUICES: JUST squeeze a little lime, lemon, or orange juice into almost any fish, bean, or chicken dish, and you'll be amazed at the extra burst of flavor. For cold dishes, add a teaspoon or so of juice as you're mixing it up. For hot dishes, squeeze the juice in toward the end of your cooking time.

DRIED FRUIT: SOME kids won't eat dried fruit because of the texture, but it's so healthy and such a great flavor booster, I encourage you to experiment. Try adding dried apricots, cranberries, currants, or blueberries to your foods. Really, you can work dried fruit into almost any recipe, from salads and muffins to stews and cookies. Soften the dried fruit in water before cooking with it.

DRIED MUSHROOMS: GROCERY stores these days have lots of dried mushrooms to choose from; I love adding dried shiitake and porcini mushrooms to pizza, soups, meatballs, or almost anything else for a little extra flavor and texture.

SUN-DRIED TOMATOES: THESE are especially great to use if tomatoes are out of season, because tomatoes are so nutritious. Sun-dried tomatoes can be softened in hot water for fifteen minutes and added to pesto, salads, or spreads for a great tangy flavor—and an extra burst of nutrition.

EXTRA LEAN KIDS

WHEN IT'S TIME to prepare a meal, teenagers can often take on the recipes—my meals are that simple and quick to prepare! Even the youngest members of the family can participate in the plan by doing these easy chores:

- ▶ FETCH FOODS from the pantry or refrigerator
- ▶ WASH FRUITS and veggies
- ▶ MEASURE INGREDIENTS
- ▶ STIR THINGS in a bowl
- ▶ SPREAD OR layer ingredients in pans
- ▶ SET THE timer and check it
- ▶ WASH OR dry dishes

KITCHEN SAFETY FOR KIDS

- ▶ SUPERVISE CHILDREN closely, especially when they're using knives or appliances
- ▶ TURN POT handles toward the inside of the stovetop

- ► KEEP ALL flammable clothing and objects away from flame and heat
- ► KEEP ELECTRICAL appliances away from water
- ► ROLL UP sleeves and tie back long hair
- ► SCRUB ALL kitchen tools that have come into contact with raw meat, poultry, fish, or eggs
- ► CLEAN UP spills as you go to prevent accidents
- ► ALWAYS USE dry pot holders to grab hot oven racks or utensils

KID-FRIENDLY KITCHEN ITEMS
- ► PLASTIC MIXING bowls and measuring cups
- ► CHILD-SIZE APRON
- ► METAL WHISKS
- ► WOODEN SPOONS
- ► RUBBER SPATULAS
- ► TOWELS WITH fun designs
- ► BRIGHT SPONGES
- ► EASY-TO-SET KITCHEN timer

Don't be discouraged if your diet isn't perfect, especially at first. Even the healthiest, most dedicated athletes and actors stray toward unhealthy meals occasionally, and everyone loves birthday cake. What you want to focus on is getting back on track as soon as possible, rather than letting unhealthy habits snowball and become persistent bad behaviors. Wake up the next morning and refocus yourself and your family on your goal of eating *Extra Lean*.

Remember, too, that your behavior and attitude toward food affect everyone else in your family. If you do have a bad meal or overindulge, and then return to solid nutritional foods, you're showing your family that it's possible to veer off course and then have the self-control to get back on track. That's a great message to send to your children not just about food but also about most things in life.

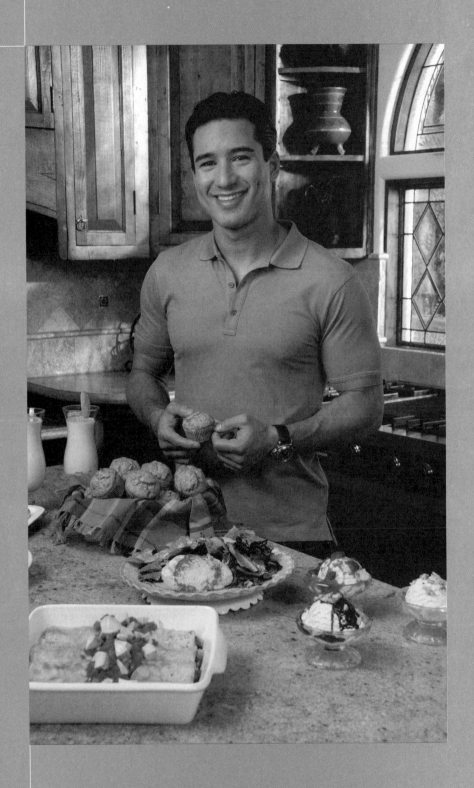

the
five-week
meal plan

AFTER FACTORING IN the basic principles behind *Extra Lean* to understand your and your family's metabolism, preparing your kitchen as well as your family for your new approach to food and *Extra Lean* living, and maintaining your short- and long-term health goals through everyday decisions about food, the focus can now be on the quick, healthy, and delicious meals. The foods that make up the five-week meal plan are based on a balance of 50 percent carbs, 25 percent protein, and 25 percent fat per day, properly portioned to keep each member of your family satisfied, and frequent enough throughout the day to keep the metabolism running high.

Of course, there will be some days when you might not hit the exact amount for each nutrient, and that's fine. There will also be slight variations in those proportions; for instance, a hungry teenager who plays soccer every day after school really does need a higher dose of carbohydrates to fuel his body, while parents who sit at their computers all day need to be extra conservative about carbohydrates in order to prevent undesired weight gain. With the meal plan, though, you and your family will never have a day when you're going overboard on carbs or undershooting protein or skipping on the healthy fats.

These meals were designed for busy families and households and with the idea that variety, freshness, taste, and health do not have to be sacrificed because of hectic schedules and the number of people to feed. That's because the recipes are not only full of flavor and metabolism-boosting foods but also require basic preparation and can be completed in twenty minutes or fewer. Also, the Double Duty option featured each week provides two meal variations for the different palates in the household using the same ingredients, and the preparation highlights allow you to plan ahead. Finally, you'll find lots of exciting new recipes to try here, as well as family favorites like tacos, macaroni casseroles, and hamburgers that are actually *good* for you.

You and your family will see food in a different way when you start preparing and cooking these meals. The meal plan will show you how clean, wholesome, and delicious foods can increase your metabolism, promote healthy eating for life, and maintain the health benefits that come from *Extra Lean* living.

GROCERY LIST

▶ **Produce**

- ☐ Strawberries: 3 quarts
- ☐ Bananas: 8
- ☐ Grapes: 2 pounds
- ☐ Apples: 12
- ☐ Celery: 1 bunch
- ☐ Cilantro: 1 bunch
- ☐ Lettuce (mixed greens or a combination of romaine and green leaf lettuces): 4 heads
- ☐ Baby carrots: 1 pound bag
- ☐ Cucumber (Kirby or English): 4
- ☐ Tomato (or cherry tomatoes): 3 medium or 1 container cherry tomatoes
- ☐ Garlic: 1 head
- ☐ Ginger root: 1 piece
- ☐ Sweet potatoes: 4 small
- ☐ Broccoli: 1¼ pounds
- ☐ Zucchini: 1 pound
- ☐ Red onions: 3
- ☐ Bell pepper: 5 red and 1 any color
- ☐ Limes: 3
- ☐ Lemons: 2
- ☐ Avocados: 2
- ☐ Orange juice: 2 half-gallon containers

▶ **Dairy & Eggs**

- ☐ Eggs: 1½ dozen
- ☐ Skim milk: 1 gallon
- ☐ Nonfat Greek yogurt: 3 large (17.6 ounce) tubs
- ☐ Unsalted butter
- ☐ String cheese: 1 package (of at least 8)
- ☐ Crumbled blue cheese: ¼ pound
- ☐ Shredded part-skim mozzarella: 1 8-ounce bag
- ☐ Provolone cheese: ¼ pound
- ☐ Sliced low fat cheese: 1½ pounds (24 slices)
- ☐ Grated Parmesan cheese

▶ **Bakery**

- ☐ Multigrain bread: 1 loaf
- ☐ Whole wheat bread: 1 loaf
- ☐ Whole wheat English muffins: 2 packages
- ☐ Whole wheat flour tortilla: 1 package (of 8)
- ☐ Whole wheat rolls: 4
- ☐ Corn tortillas: 1 package (of 8)

▶ **Meat & Deli and Seafood**

- ☐ Chicken breast (boneless, skinless): 2½ pounds

GROCERY LIST

- Low sodium turkey breast: 1 pound
- Ground chicken sausage: 1 12-ounce package
- Frozen large shrimp: 1 pound
- Tilapia: 4 pieces (about 1¼ pounds)
- Flank steak or London broil: 1 pound
- Ground turkey breast (or premade burgers): 1 pound
- Pizza dough: 24 ounces
- Hummus: 2 16-ounce tubs

▶ **Frozen**

- Whole grain waffles

▶ **Grocery & Pantry Items**

- Whole grain cereal: 2 boxes
- Rolled oats: 1 small canister
- Granola: 1 package
- Almonds: 1 6-ounce package
- Whole wheat pretzels: 1 12-ounce bag
- Whole grain pasta (suggested: penne): 1 12-ounce box
- Brown rice
- All-purpose flour
- Baking soda
- Baking powder
- Unsweetened cocoa powder
- Cornstarch
- Granulated sugar
- Miniature chocolate chips: 1 small bag
- Reduced sodium soy sauce

- Barbecue sauce
- Mustard
- Chili sauce
- Maple syrup
- Fruit spread
- Natural peanut butter
- Balsamic vinaigrette
- Rice vinegar
- Vanilla extract
- Agave nectar
- Unsweetened applesauce
- Salsa
- Canned tuna (in water): 6 15-ounce cans
- Mayonnaise
- Canned crushed tomatoes: 1 28-ounce can
- Canned black beans: 1 15-ounce can
- Olive oil
- Canola oil
- Nonstick cooking spray
- Ground cinnamon
- Ground cumin
- Kosher salt
- Black pepper
- Chili powder

HIGHLIGHTS

Prep Day on Sunday

- ▶ Grill 2 pounds of chicken breast for Sunday night dinner and lunches on Monday and Thursday
- ▶ Cook a total of 2.5 cups dry brown rice. This will yield 7 cups of cooked rice—3 cups for Sunday night dinner and 4 more cups for Wednesday night dinner

Meatless Monday option for Week 1: whole wheat pasta with mixed vegetables—topped with olive oil and Parmesan cheese. So simple and yummy—a trick is to save a bit of the pasta cooking liquid to toss with the pasta, veggies, and cheese.

Whole grain cereal recommendations: Bran Flakes, Kashi Go Lean, or Nature's Path Multigrain Flakes

Fruits for the week: apples, bananas, strawberries, and grapes (there will always be a high-fiber berry choice each week.)

Friday night's "make your own takeout" is pizza—making your own will save hundreds of calories.

Always use natural peanut butter—ingredients should be only peanuts and salt.

Freeze leftovers of bread, rolls, English muffins, and brownies—they will keep well in a freezer-safe bag for up to three months.

- ■ microwave the sweet potato (Tuesday night dinner)

- ■ use frozen raw shrimp for Wednesday night's stir fry—all you have to do is defrost the shrimp in a bowl of water for 10 minutes and they are ready to use

TIME SAVER
TIPS

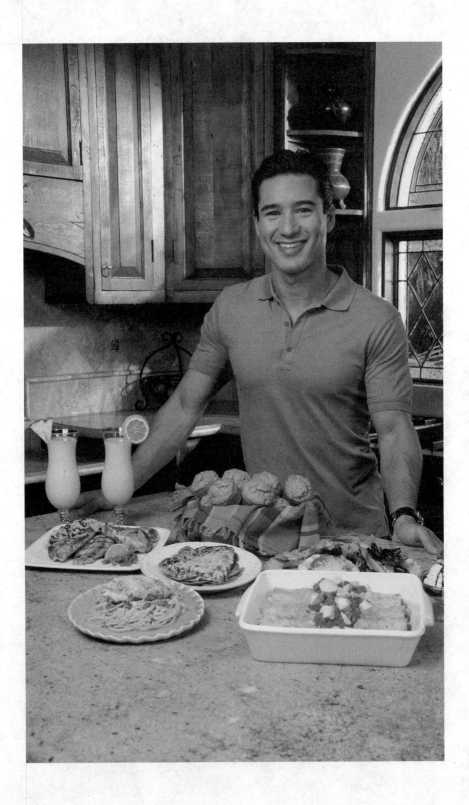

BREAKFAST

▶ **6 fl oz orange juice**

▶ **Cinnamon-Banana French Toast**
SERVES: 4

2 bananas, sliced
4 tablespoons maple syrup
1 teaspoon cinnamon, divided
4 large eggs
1 cup skim milk
1 teaspoon vanilla extract
4 teaspoons unsalted butter
8 slices multigrain bread

1. In a small bowl combine bananas and maple syrup; sprinkle with ½ teaspoon cinnamon, mix and set aside. In medium bowl, combine eggs, milk, vanilla, and remaining cinnamon, whisk well. Heat 1 teaspoon of butter in a nonstick skillet or griddle over medium heat. Dunk two slices of bread into egg mixture and transfer to hot pan. Cook for 2–3 minutes per side until golden brown. Repeat for remaining slices of bread, using an additional teaspoon of butter for each batch. Transfer to a plate and top with banana mixture.

Check labels and spend the extra money on the real stuff. Some maple syrups are colored sugar syrups in disguise

Total Calories: 452
Total Fat: 8.5g
Saturated Fat: 3g
Carbohydrate: 80g
Protein: 16g
Sodium: 355mg
Cholesterol: 117mg
Fiber: 10g

NUTRIENT INTAKE:

Carbs 69%

Protein 14%

Fat 17%

LUNCH

▶ **Turkey & Cheese with Hummus:** 4 slices low sodium turkey breast with 1 slice low fat cheese, lettuce, tomato, and 2 tablespoons hummus on a whole wheat English muffin

Hummus is filled with healthy fats and protein, a healthier and more satisfying alternative to mayo

Calories: 362	**NUTRIENT INTAKE:**
Total Fat: 11g	Carbs 37%
Saturated Fat: 4g	Protein 36%
Carbohydrate: 33g	Fat 27%
Protein: 33g	
Sodium: 80mg	
Cholesterol: 45mg	
Fiber: 7g	

SNACK

▶ **1 cup grapes**

Calories: 110	**NUTRIENT INTAKE:**
Total Fat: 0g	Carbs 94%
Saturated Fat: 0g	Protein 4%
Carbohydrate: 29g	Fat 2%
Protein: 1g	
Sodium: 3mg	
Cholesterol: 0g	
Fiber: 1.5g	

DINNER

Extra Prep:

- grill 1 extra pound of chicken breast
- cook 2.5 cups (dry) brown rice to make enough for the week

▶ **BBQ Chicken with Rice & Beans**

SERVES: 4

1 pound boneless, skinless chicken breast (4 pieces)
2 tablespoons canola oil, divided
Salt and pepper
¼ cup barbecue sauce
1 lime
2 cloves garlic, minced
1 bell pepper, finely chopped
½ teaspoon ground cumin
1 (15-oz) can black beans, rinsed and drained
3 cups cooked brown rice (1 cup dry yields 3 cups cooked)
½ cup fresh cilantro, chopped

Canned beans are a huge time-saver; make sure to rinse them well to remove some of the sodium.

1. Heat grill or grill pan to medium-high. Season chicken breast with 4 teaspoons canola oil, salt, and pepper. Place on grill and cook for 6–7 minutes per side. Brush each side with barbecue sauce and cook for an additional 2–3 minutes

or until cooked through. Transfer to a plate and squeeze fresh lime juice over the top.

2. While the chicken is cooking, prepare the rice and beans. Heat remaining oil in a large skillet, add garlic, bell pepper, cumin, and ¼ teaspoon salt—sauté for 2–3 minutes. Add black beans and brown rice and continue to cook until rice is warm. Mix in cilantro and serve.

▶ Cucumber Salad

SERVES: 4

4 cups thinly sliced cucumber (3 to 4 large cucumbers—
Kirby or English hothouse recommended)
½ teaspoon kosher salt
2 tablespoons rice vinegar
Thinly sliced red onion to taste
Black pepper to taste

1. Place sliced cucumber in a large bowl and season with salt. Toss well and set aside for 5–10 minutes to allow cucumber to release some of its water—drain well. Add vinegar, red onion, and black pepper; toss well and serve.

Total Calories: 521
Total Fat: 11g
Saturated Fat: 2g
Carbohydrate: 51g
Protein: 52g
Sodium: 320mg
Cholesterol: 120mg
Fiber: 6.5g

NUTRIENT INTAKE:

Carbs 40%
Protein 41%
Fat 19%

NUTRITION FOR THE DAY

Total Calories: 1446
Total Fat: 30.5g
Saturated Fat: 10g
Carbohydrate: 193g
Protein: 103g
Sodium: 1589mg
Cholesterol: 188mg
Fiber: 25g

NUTRIENT INTAKE:

Carbs 53%
Protein 28%
Fat 19%

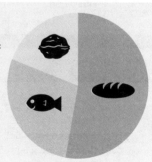

1 MONDAY

BREAKFAST

- ▶ 1½ cups whole grain cereal
- ▶ 1 cup skim milk
- ▶ ½ cup sliced strawberries

Total Calories: 311
Total Fat: 2g
Saturated Fat: 0.5g
Carbohydrate: 67g
Protein: 15g
Sodium: 400mg
Cholesterol: 5mg
Fiber: 12g

NUTRIENT INTAKE:

Carbs 77%
Protein 17%
Fat 6%

LUNCH

Double Duty Option:

- ▶ **Cobb Salad with grilled chicken:** 3 cups mixed greens topped with 4 oz grilled chicken, ⅓ cup diced avocado, 1 tablespoon crumbled blue cheese, chopped tomato, and 2 teaspoons olive oil & lemon juice to taste

OR

- ▶ **Grilled Chicken Wraps:** grilled chicken with mustard, lettuce, tomato, and cheese in a whole wheat tortilla

Calories: 480
Total Fat: 29g
Saturated Fat: 8.5g
Carbohydrate: 14g
Protein: 42g
Sodium: 306mg
Cholesterol: 107mg
Fiber: 7.5g

NUTRIENT INTAKE:

Carbs 12%
Protein 34%
Fat 54%

SNACK

- ▶ 1 string cheese
- ▶ 15 almonds

Calories: 184
Total Fat: 15g
Saturated Fat: 4.5g
Carbohydrate: 5g
Protein: 11g
Sodium: 220mg
Cholesterol: 20mg
Fiber: 2g

NUTRIENT INTAKE:

Carbs 9%
Protein 22%
Fat 69%

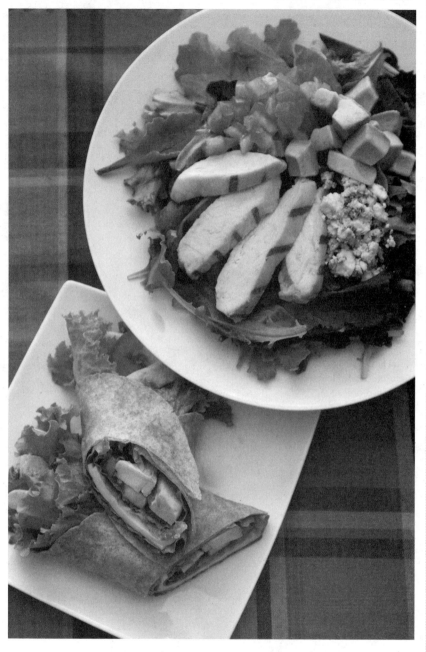

Double Duty: Cobb Salad with Grilled Chicken and Grilled Chicken Wrap

DINNER

▶ **Pasta with Vegetables:** 1½ cups cooked whole wheat penne topped with 1 cup mixed vegetables, 2 teaspoons olive oil, and 2 tablespoons grated Parmesan cheese

LEFTOVER TIP: Toss whole wheat pasta with chicken, beans, bell peppers, broccoli, and balsamic vinaigrette

Calories: 526
Total Fat: 14g
Saturated Fat: 3g
Carbohydrate: 84g
Protein: 23g
Sodium: 232mg
Cholesterol: 9mg
Fiber: 17g

NUTRIENT INTAKE:

Carbs 61%

Protein 16%

Fat 23%

NUTRITION FOR THE DAY

Calories: 1500
Total Fat: 60g
Saturated Fat: 14.5g
Carbohydrate: 170g
Protein: 90g
Sodium: 1328mg
Cholesterol: 141mg
Fiber: 39g

NUTRIENT INTAKE:

Carbs 45%

Protein 25%

Fat 30%

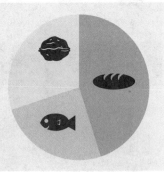

BREAKFAST

▶ 2 tablespoons natural peanut butter

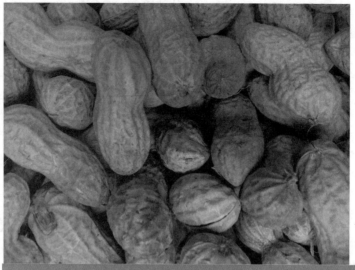

Natural peanut butter has no added sugars.
Ingredients should just be peanuts.

▶ 1 slice whole wheat bread
▶ 1 apple

Double Duty Option:

- Swap out bread for a whole grain waffle

Calories: 363
Total Fat: 18g
Saturated Fat: 3g
Carbohydrate: 39g
Protein: 11g
Sodium: 166mg
Cholesterol: 0mg
Fiber: 12g

NUTRIENT INTAKE:

Carbs 43%
Protein 12%
Fat 45%

LUNCH

▶ 1 oz whole wheat pretzels

TUESDAY

► **Tuna Salad with Grapes** on a whole wheat English muffin
SERVES: 4

Grapes jazz up this tuna salad—they add sweetness and crunch!

3 5-ounce cans of tuna, packed in water
2 tablespoons mayonnaise
2 tablespoons nonfat Greek yogurt
½ cup chopped celery
1 cup grapes, halved
Black pepper to taste

1. Combine ingredients in a bowl and mix gently with a fork to combine.

  **make double batch of the recipe for lunch on Saturday

Total Calories: 438
Total Fat: 9g
Saturated Fat: 1g
Carbohydrate: 56g
Protein: 39g
Sodium: 795mg
Cholesterol: 49mg
Fiber: 5g

NUTRIENT INTAKE:

Carbs 49%
Protein 34%
Fat 17%

SNACK

► **10 baby carrots**
► **½ cup hummus**

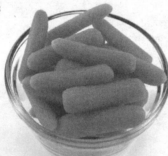

Calories: 175
Total Fat: 6g
Saturated Fat: 0g
Carbohydrate: 24g
Protein: 5g
Sodium: 538mg
Cholesterol: 0mg
Fiber: 6g

NUTRIENT INTAKE:

Carbs 57%
Protein 11%
Fat 32%

DINNER

► **1 piece tilapia (about 5 oz) sautéed in 2 teaspoons olive oil**

> **Tilapia** is a very user-friendly fish. It's mild, protein-packed, and cooks up in minutes.

► **2 cups broccoli roasted with 2 teaspoons extra virgin olive oil**
► **1 small baked sweet potato topped with 2 tablespoons nonfat Greek yogurt**

Calories: 482
Total Fat: 18.5g
Saturated Fat: 3g
Carbohydrate: 45g
Protein: 45g
Sodium: 212mg
Cholesterol: 92mg
Fiber: 8.5g

NUTRIENT INTAKE:

Carbs 30%
Protein 36%
Fat 34%

NUTRITION FOR THE DAY

Calories: 1457
Total Fat: 52g
Saturated Fat: 7g
Carbohydrate: 156g
Protein: 100g
Sodium: 1711mg
Cholesterol: 141mg
Fiber: 30g

NUTRIENT INTAKE:

Carbs 45%

Protein 27%

Fat 28%

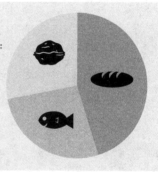

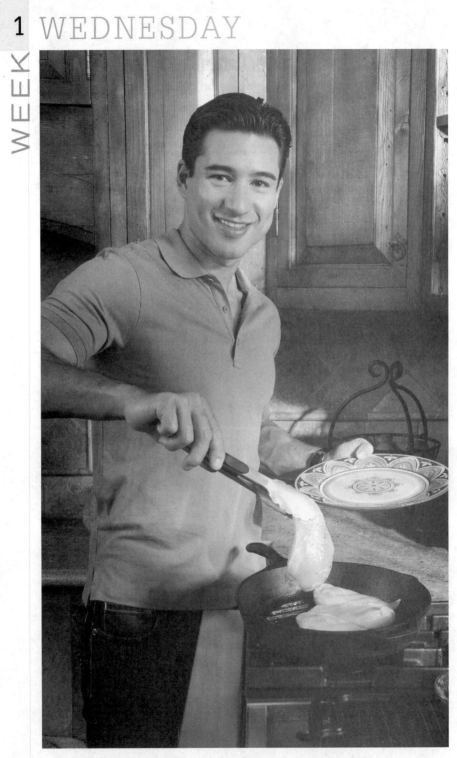

BREAKFAST

- ► 1½ cups whole grain cereal
- ► 1 cup skim milk
- ► ½ cup sliced strawberries

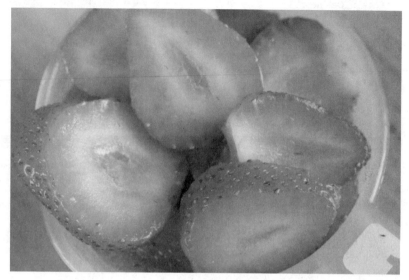

Calories: 311
Total Fat: 2g
Saturated Fat: 0.5g
Carbohydrate: 67g
Protein: 15g
Sodium: 400mg
Cholesterol: 5mg
Fiber: 12g

NUTRIENT INTAKE:

Carbs 77%
Protein 17%
Fat 6%

LUNCH

- ► **Turkey & cheese roll-ups:** 4 slices low sodium turkey breast with 2 slices low fat cheese
- ► **1 oz whole grain pretzels**
- ► **2 cups mixed greens topped with 1 tablespoon balsamic vinaigrette**

Calories: 383
Total Fat: 18g
Saturated Fat: 7.5g
Carbohydrate: 28g
Protein: 28g
Sodium: 803mg
Cholesterol: 50mg
Fiber: 3g

NUTRIENT INTAKE:

Carbs 29%
Protein 29%
Fat 42%

SNACK

▸ **1 string cheese**
▸ **15 almonds**

Calories: 184
Total Fat: 15g
Saturated Fat: 4.5g
Carbohydrate: 5g
Protein: 11g
Sodium: 220mg
Cholesterol: 20mg
Fiber: 2g

NUTRIENT INTAKE:

Carbs 9%

Protein 22%

Fat 69%

DINNER

▸ **1 cup cooked brown rice**

▸ **Ginger-Garlic Shrimp**
SERVES: 4

Stir-fry makes a quick and easy weeknight dinner—save even more time by chopping the ingredients and making the sauce ahead of time

For the sauce:
2 tablespoons reduced sodium soy sauce
½ cup water or chicken stock
1 tablespoon sugar
2 teaspoons cornstarch
Chili sauce to taste, such as Sriracha (optional)

1 tablespoon canola oil
3 cloves garlic, minced
1 tablespoon minced fresh ginger root
1 pound raw large shrimp (peeled and deveined)
2 large red or orange bell pepper, sliced
1 pound zucchini, sliced

1. Combine sauce ingredients in a measuring cup, whisk well to incorporate corn-starch and set aside.
2. Heat oil in a large skillet or wok over high heat. Add garlic, ginger, and shrimp and sauté for 2–3 minutes. Add peppers and zucchini and toss well. Add sauce and continue to toss and cook for 5–6 minutes until vegetables are slightly tender.

Double Duty Option:

- Thread shrimp and veggies onto skewers, baste with soy sauce, and grill. Serve over brown rice.

LEFTOVER TIP: Grill up some shrimp and add to a salad or combine with cooked rice, black beans, and salsa in a whole wheat tortilla.

Total Calories: 414
Total Fat: 7g
Saturated Fat: 1g
Carbohydrate: 57g
Protein: 30g
Sodium: 497mg
Cholesterol: 172mg
Fiber: 6g

NUTRIENT INTAKE:

Carbs 55%

Protein 29%

Fat 16%

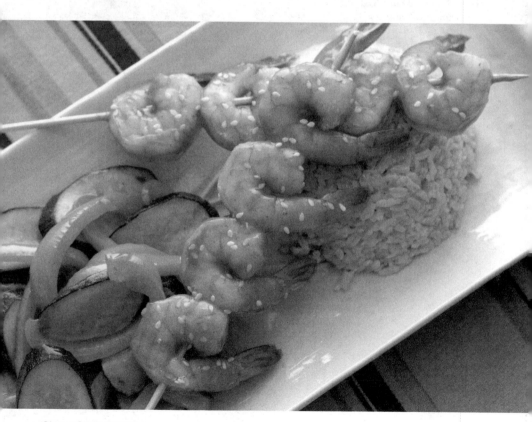

Ginger-Garlic Shrimp

WEDNESDAY

DESSERT

▶ **Fruit Parfaits:** ¾ cup nonfat Greek yogurt layered in a glass with ½ cup each sliced strawberries and bananas. Top with 2 tablespoons granola.

Calories: 216
Total Fat: 1g
Saturated Fat: 0g
Carbohydrate: 36g
Protein: 18g
Sodium: 64mg
Cholesterol: 0mg
Fiber: 4g

NUTRIENT INTAKE:

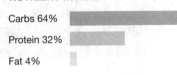

Carbs 64%

Protein 32%

Fat 4%

NUTRITION FOR THE DAY

Calories: 1508
Total Fat: 43.5g
Saturated Fat: 13.5g
Carbohydrate: 192g
Protein: 101g
Sodium: 2157mg
Cholesterol: 247mg
Fiber: 28g

NUTRIENT INTAKE:

Carbs 49%

Protein 26%

Fat 25%

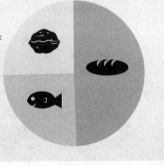

BREAKFAST

▶ 1 cup cooked oatmeal topped with ⅓ cup granola
▶ 6 fl oz orange juice

Calories: 459
Total Fat: 5g
Saturated Fat: 0.5g
Carbohydrate: 95g
Protein: 11g
Sodium: 366mg
Cholesterol: 0mg
Fiber: 7g

NUTRIENT INTAKE:

Carbs 81%

Protein 10%

Fat 9%

LUNCH

Double Duty Option:

▶ **Chicken Salsa Wraps:** grilled chicken with cheese, salsa, and lettuce in a whole wheat tortilla

OR

▶ **Grilled Chicken Salad:** 3 cups mixed greens topped with 4 oz grilled chicken, ⅓ cup diced avocado, 1 tablespoon salsa, 2 tablespoons shredded cheese, chopped tomato, and 2 teaspoons olive oil & lime juice to taste

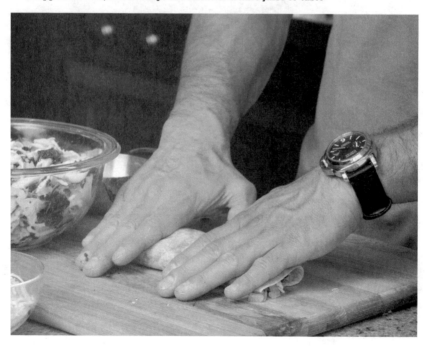

Calories: 470
Total Fat: 28g
Saturated Fat: 7.5g
Carbohydrate: 14g
Protein: 42g
Sodium: 306mg
Cholesterol: 107mg
Fiber: 7.5g

NUTRIENT INTAKE:

Carbs 12%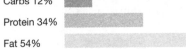
Protein 34%
Fat 54%

SNACK

- ▸ 1 apple
- ▸ 1 tablespoon peanut butter

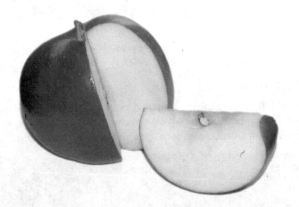

Calories: 177
Total Fat: 9g
Saturated Fat: 1.5g
Carbohydrate: 22g
Protein: 4g
Sodium: 16mg
Cholesterol: 0mg
Fiber: 5g

NUTRIENT INTAKE:

Carbs 48%
Protein 9%
Fat 43%

DINNER

- ▸ **4 oz turkey burgers served on whole wheat rolls:** Get premade burgers or mix 1 pound ground turkey breast with ¼ cup finely chopped onion and 2 tablespoons mustard (makes 4 burgers)
- ▸ **2 cups mixed greens topped with 1 tablespoon each balsamic vinaigrette and** crumbled blue cheese

Calories: 442
Total Fat: 16g
Saturated Fat: 6g
Carbohydrate: 34g
Protein: 40g
Sodium: 962mg
Cholesterol: 91mg
Fiber: 5g

NUTRIENT INTAKE:

Carbs 31%
Protein 36%
Fat 33%

NUTRITION FOR THE DAY

Calories: 1558
Total Fat: 58.5g
Saturated Fat: 15g
Carbohydrate: 166g
Protein: 97g
Sodium: 1650mg
Cholesterol: 198mg
Fiber: 25g

NUTRIENT INTAKE:

Carbs 45%

Protein 25%

Fat 30%

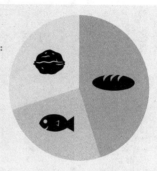

BREAKFAST

▶ Rise & Shine Smoothie

SERVES: 2

2 bananas, chopped
12 fl oz orange juice
1 cup nonfat Greek yogurt
Water and ice as desired (optional)

1. Place ingredients in a blender and blend until smooth.

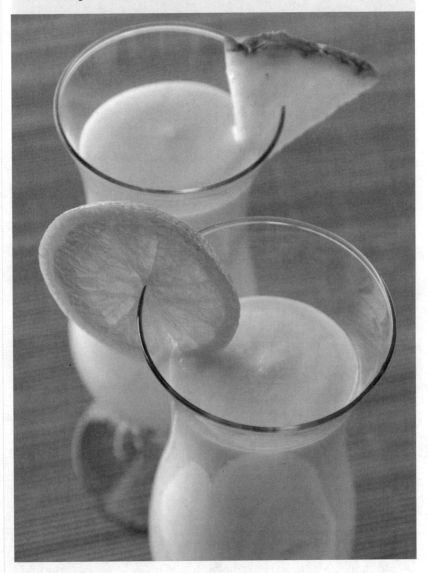

Total Calories: 274
Total Fat: 0g
Saturated Fat: 0g
Carbohydrate: 58g
Protein: 13g
Sodium: 44mg
Cholesterol: 0mg
Fiber: 4g

NUTRIENT INTAKE:

Carbs 80%
Protein 18%
Fat 2%

LUNCH

▶ **Peanut Butter & Jam:** 2 slices whole wheat bread topped with 2 tablespoons peanut butter and 1 tablespoon fruit spread

When buying fruit spread, check labels and get one made with real fruit and sweetened with fruit juice to cut back on added sugars.

▶ **8 fl oz skim milk**

Calories: 497
Total Fat: 19.5g
Saturated Fat: 3g
Carbohydrate: 56g
Protein: 23g
Sodium: 431mg
Cholesterol: 5mg
Fiber: 11g

NUTRIENT INTAKE

Carbs 46%
Protein 19%
Fat 35%

SNACK

▶ **10 baby carrots**
▶ **½ cup hummus**

Calories: 175
Total Fat: 6g
Saturated Fat: 0g
Carbohydrate: 24g
Protein: 5g
Sodium: 538mg
Cholesterol: 0mg
Fiber: 6g

NUTRIENT INTAKE:

Carbs 57%
Protein 11%
Fat 32%

DINNER

- ▶ 2 cups mixed greens
- ▶ 1 tablespoon balsamic vinaigrette

- ▶ **"Take-out night": Sausage & Pepper Pizza**

MAKES: 12 SLICES (2 slices per serving. save some slices for the following week)

*Who doesn't love pizza—homemade versions have much less grease!
Stop by your local pizzeria for affordable and delicious fresh dough and
for fresh tomato sauce, take half of a 28-ounce can of crushed tomatoes
and season with ½ teaspoon salt, ½ teaspoon garlic, and 1 tablespoon
olive oil.*

24-ounce piece of pizza dough (store-bought or homemade)
1 cup tomato sauce
6 ounces ground chicken sausage, cooked in a nonstick skillet for 5–6 minutes, set
    aside to cool slightly
4 oz provolone cheese
½ cup shredded part-skim mozzarella cheese
½ red onion, thinly sliced
1 large bell pepper, thinly sliced into rings

1. Preheat oven to 450 degrees F. On a lightly floured surface, roll out pizza dough
   and gently stretch it on a pizza pan or baking sheet. Top dough with tomato
   sauce, sausage, and cheese. Add onion and peppers and bake for 20 minutes
   or until crust is golden and cheese is melted and bubbly. Allow to rest for 10
   minutes before slicing.

Total Calories: 566
Total Fat: 24g
Saturated Fat: 5.5g
Carbohydrate: 58g
Protein: 26g
Sodium: 1428mg
Cholesterol: 57mg
Fiber: 4g

NUTRIENT INTAKE:

Carbs 42%
Protein 19%
Fat 39%

NUTRITION FOR THE DAY

Calories: 1513
Total Fat: 50g
Saturated Fat: 13g
Carbohydrate: 196g
Protein: 68g
Sodium: 2340mg
Cholesterol: 161mg
Fiber: 25g

NUTRIENT INTAKE:

Carbs 52%
Protein 20%
Fat 28%

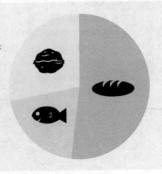

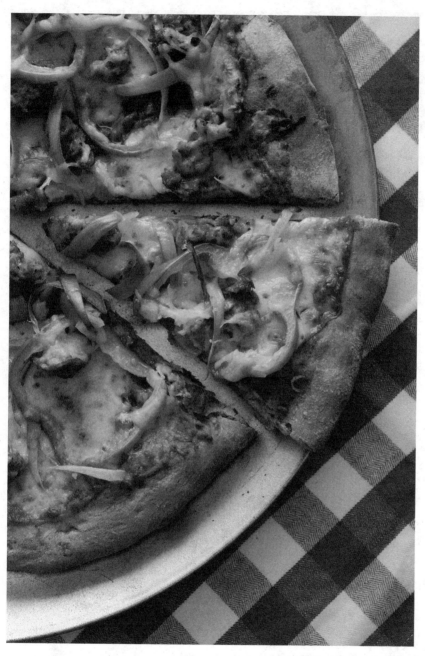

BREAKFAST

▶ **2 eggs, scrambled with ½ cup vegetables**

LEFTOVER TIP: Try scrambled eggs with vegetables and low fat cheese for dinner—add a slice or two of whole grain toast and a small salad to complete the meal

▶ **1 toasted whole wheat English muffin**
▶ **1 banana**

Calories: 395
Total Fat: 11.5g
Saturated Fat: 3.5g
Carbohydrate: 56g
Protein: 20g
Sodium: 374mg
Cholesterol: 423mg
Fiber: 7g

NUTRIENT INTAKE:

Carbs 54%

Protein 20%

Fat 26%

LUNCH

▶ **1 cup strawberries**
▶ **Tuna Melts:** Tuna Salad with Grapes (see Tuesday's lunch for the recipe) on top of one slice of whole wheat bread. Add a slice of tomato and low fat cheese. Place in the oven for 5 minutes or until cheese is melted.

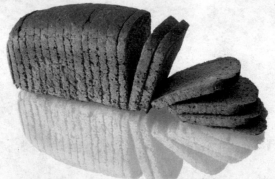

Calories: 429
Total Fat: 14.5g
Saturated Fat: 4g
Carbohydrate: 36g
Protein: 42g
Sodium: 768mg
Cholesterol: 64mg
Fiber: 8g

NUTRIENT INTAKE:

Carbs 32%

Protein 39%

Fat 29%

SNACK

▶ **1 apple**

Calories: 72
Total Fat: 0g
Saturated Fat: 0g
Carbohydrate: 19g
Protein: 0g
Sodium: 1mg
Cholesterol: 0g
Fiber: 3g

NUTRIENT INTAKE:

Carbs 96%

Protein 2%

Fat 2%

DINNER

▶ **Steak Fajitas**
SERVES: 4

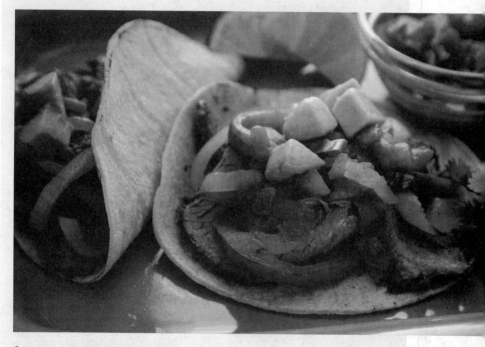

2 teaspoons canola oil
1 large onion, thinly sliced
2 large bell peppers, sliced
¼ teaspoon kosher salt
¼ teaspoon chili powder
1 pound piece flank steak or London broil, grilled and thinly sliced

8 corn tortillas, warmed

1 cup diced avocado
1 cup salsa
Lime wedges

1. Heat oil in a large skillet, add onions and peppers. Season vegetables with salt and chili powder and sauté for 3–4 minutes. To assemble fajitas, place steak in corn tortilla and top with onion and pepper mixture, avocado, salsa, and freshly squeezed lime juice.

Calories: 486
Total Fat: 20g
Saturated Fat: 5.5g
Carbohydrate: 42g
Protein: 37g
Sodium: 336mg
Cholesterol: 62mg
Fiber: 10.5g

NUTRIENT INTAKE

Carbs 34%

Protein 30%

Fat 36%

DESSERT

▶ Dark Chocolate Brownies

MAKES 9 BROWNIES

This recipe makes 9 large brownies—split one and save half the calories!

Nonstick cooking spray
½ cup all-purpose flour
½ cup unsweetened cocoa powder
¼ teaspoon baking powder
⅛ teaspoon baking soda
⅛ teaspoon kosher salt

4 tablespoons unsalted butter, melted
¼ cup agave nectar

Agave nectar is another natural sweetener to add to your pantry. It's more sweet than honey, so you'll use less.

½ cup unsweetened applesauce
½ cup sugar
2 tablespoons canola oil

1 teaspoon vanilla extract
2 large eggs

½ cup miniature chocolate chips

> **Use applesauce** to help cut the fat in baking.

1. Spray a 9x9 square baking dish with cooking spray and set aside. Combine flour, cocoa, baking powder, baking soda, and salt in a bowl and set aside. Melt butter in a medium saucepan. Transfer hot butter to a large glass bowl. Whisk in agave, applesauce, sugar, canola oil, and vanilla. Whisk in eggs one at a time. Transfer mixture to prepared baking dish. Sprinkle with chocolate chips and bake for 25–30 minutes or until a cake tester comes out clean from the center. Cool for at least 20 minutes before cutting into squares.

Calories: 194
Total Fat: 10g
Saturated Fat: 4g
Carbohydrate: 27g
Protein: 3g
Sodium: 64mg
Cholesterol: 61mg
Fiber: 2g

NUTRIENT INTAKE:

Carbs 51%
Protein 6%
Fat 43%

NUTRITION FOR THE DAY

Calories: 1578
Total Fat: 56g
Saturated Fat: 17.5g
Carbohydrate: 180mg
Protein: 103g
Sodium: 1543mg
Cholesterol: 610mg
Fiber: 31g

NUTRIENT INTAKE:

Carbs 45%
Protein 25%
Fat 30%

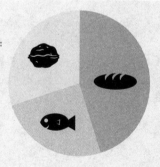

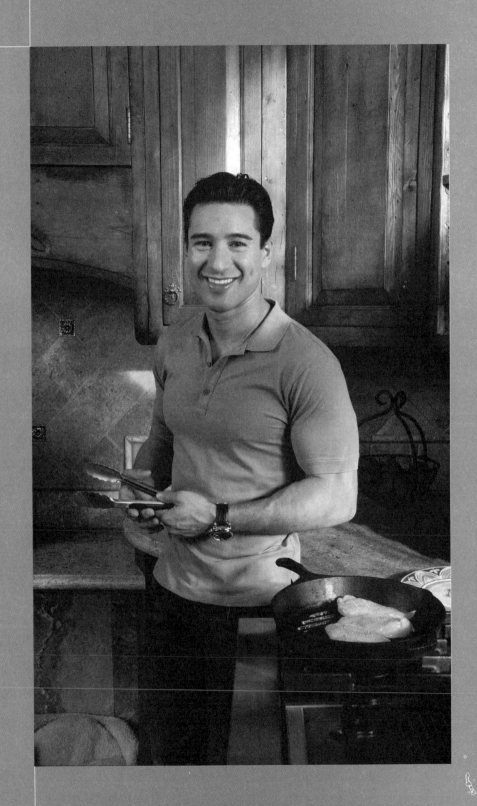

GROCERY LIST

▶ **Produce**

- ☐ Pineapples: 2
- ☐ Oranges: 4
- ☐ Apples: 14
- ☐ Grapes: 2¾ pounds
- ☐ Blueberries: 2 pints
- ☐ Strawberries [fresh or frozen (unsweetened)]: 1 pint
- ☐ Orange: 1
- ☐ Celery: 1 bunch
- ☐ Parsley: 1 bunch
- ☐ Lettuce (mixed greens or a combination of romaine and green leaf lettuces): 4 heads
- ☐ Baby spinach: 1 small package
- ☐ Cucumbers: 3
- ☐ Tomatoes (or cherry tomatoes): 5 medium or 2 containers cherry tomatoes
- ☐ Garlic: 1 head
- ☐ Sweet potato: 1 medium
- ☐ Yukon gold or russet potatoes: 4 medium
- ☐ Broccoli: 1 bunch
- ☐ Red onions: 2
- ☐ Scallions: 1 bunch
- ☐ Red bell peppers: 2
- ☐ Jalapeno pepper: 1
- ☐ Poblano pepper: 2

- ☐ Lemons: 2
- ☐ Avocados: 2
- ☐ Orange juice: ½ gallon

▶ **Dairy & Eggs**

- ☐ Eggs: 2 dozen
- ☐ Skim milk: 1 gallon
- ☐ Nonfat Greek yogurt: 4 large containers
- ☐ Reduced fat (2%) Greek yogurt: 1 large container
- ☐ Nonfat fruit yogurt: 8 6-ounce containers
- ☐ Low fat plain yogurt: 1 small (6-ounce) container
- ☐ Shredded Mexican blend cheese: 1 package
- ☐ Crumbled low fat feta cheese: 6 ounces
- ☐ Swiss cheese: ½ pound
- ☐ Shredded cheddar cheese: 1 package
- ☐ Sliced low fat American, cheddar, or Swiss cheese (for sandwiches): 12 slices

▶ **Bakery**

- ☐ Whole wheat pita: 12
- ☐ Whole wheat bread: 1 loaf
- ☐ Whole wheat English muffins: 8

the five-week **meal plan**   95

- ☐ Whole wheat flour tortilla: 4
- ☐ Whole wheat hamburger rolls: 4
- ☐ Plain angel food cake: 1 cake

▶ **Meat & Deli and Seafood**

- ☐ Chicken breast (boneless, skinless): 1 pound
- ☐ Rotisserie chicken: 1
- ☐ Ground turkey breast: 1 pound
- ☐ Low sodium turkey breast: 1½ pounds
- ☐ Ground beef (90% lean): 1 pound
- ☐ Wild salmon: 1 pound
- ☐ Pork tenderloin: 1 pound
- ☐ Hummus: 1 large container

▶ **Grocery & Pantry Items**

- ☐ Whole grain cereal: 1 box
- ☐ Whole grain crackers: 1 box
- ☐ Rolled oats: 1 canister
- ☐ Slivered almonds
- ☐ Baked tortilla chips: 1 bag
- ☐ Chopped walnuts
- ☐ Quinoa
- ☐ Brown rice
- ☐ Granulated sugar
- ☐ Reduced sodium soy sauce
- ☐ Worcestershire sauce
- ☐ Dijon mustard
- ☐ Ketchup
- ☐ Low sodium chicken broth
- ☐ Maple syrup
- ☐ Fruit spread

- ☐ Natural peanut butter
- ☐ Almond butter
- ☐ Balsamic vinaigrette
- ☐ Low fat Ranch dressing
- ☐ Agave nectar
- ☐ Salsa
- ☐ Dried cranberries
- ☐ Dark beer (12 fl oz)
- ☐ Canned crushed tomatoes: 3 28-ounce cans
- ☐ Canned black beans: 1 15-ounce can
- ☐ Pinto beans: 1 15-ounce can
- ☐ Red kidney beans: 1 15-ounce can
- ☐ Pitted black olives: 1 small can
- ☐ Olive oil
- ☐ Canola oil
- ☐ Sesame oil
- ☐ Nonstick cooking spray
- ☐ Ground cinnamon
- ☐ Kosher salt
- ☐ Black pepper

HIGHLIGHTS

Prep Day on Sunday

▶ Chili will be for dinner Sunday night and Wednesday

▶ Cook quinoa and store in the fridge for Tuesday night

  • Rinse and drain quinoa well. In a saucepan, combine quinoa, water, and a pinch of salt. Bring to a boil, reduce heat, cover and simmer for 15–20 minutes, until water is absorbed and quinoa is tender. One cup dry will yield 3 cups cooked.

Meatless Monday option for Week 2: Veggie Quesadillas—whole wheat tortillas, cheese, and lots of vegetables. Veggies can be interchanged for others—meal comes together in minutes.

Whole grain cereal recommendations: Bran Flakes, Kashi Go Lean, or Nature's Path Multigrain Flakes

Fruits for the week: apples, blueberries, pineapple, oranges, strawberries (for frozen yogurt)

Friday night's "make your own takeout" is Burgers and Fries (oven fries)—no stopping at the drive-through—making your own will save hundreds of calories.

TIME SAVER TIPS

■ Make extra oatmeal—can be microwaved later in the week for breakfast in seconds

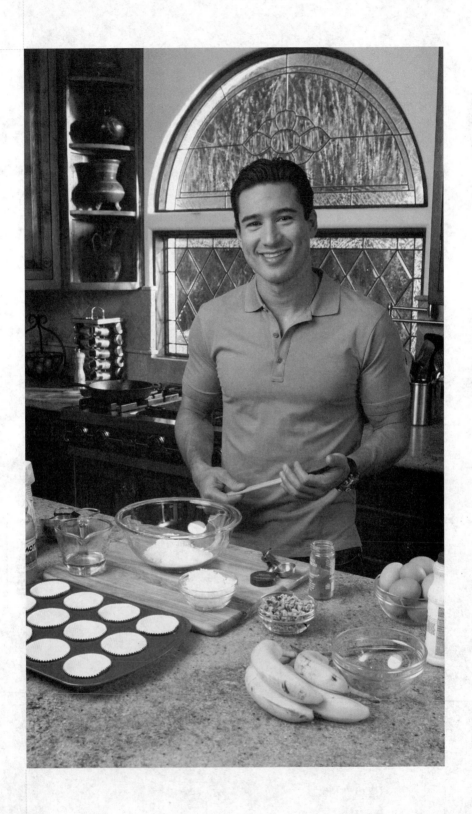

BREAKFAST

▸ 1 cup nonfat Greek yogurt topped with ¾ cup pineapple and 3 tablespoons slivered almonds

Calories: 293
Total Fat: 11g
Saturated Fat: 1g
Carbohydrate: 28g
Protein: 25g
Sodium: 86mg
Cholesterol: 0mg
Fiber: 4g

NUTRIENT INTAKE

Carbs 36%
Protein 33%
Fat 31%

LUNCH

▸ 2 slices leftover pizza from Friday night
▸ 1 orange

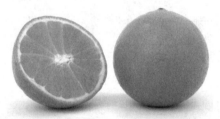

Calories: 487
Total Fat: 13.5g
Saturated Fat: 4g
Carbohydrate: 67g
Protein: 21g
Sodium: 1018mg
Cholesterol: 19mg
Fiber: 6g

NUTRIENT INTAKE:

Carbs 57%
Protein 17%
Fat 26%

SNACK

▸ 1 apple
▸ 1 tablespoon peanut or almond butter

Calories: 235
Total Fat: 10g
Saturated Fat: 1g
Carbohydrate: 13g
Protein: 4g
Sodium: 73mg
Cholesterol: 0mg
Fiber: 7g

NUTRIENT INTAKE:

Carbs 59%
Protein 6%
Fat 35%

DINNER

▸ **1 oz baked tortilla chips**

Some baked tortilla brands have as much as 50 percent less fat than regular chips: you'll save fat and calories.

▸ **2 cups mixed greens**
▸ **2 tablespoons balsamic vinaigrette**

▸ **Spicy Turkey Chili**

MAKES 8 SERVINGS

Not a huge fan of spicy? You can always dial down the heat by using less chili powder.

Spice Mix:

1 teaspoon ground cumin
2 tablespoons chili powder (or to taste)
½ teaspoon celery salt

Chili:

1 tablespoon canola oil
1 pound ground turkey breast
1 medium red onion, diced
1 red bell pepper, diced
1 jalapeno pepper, finely diced (optional)
½ cup chopped celery
3 cloves minced garlic
½ teaspoon kosher salt
½ cup chicken broth or water
1 teaspoon Worcestershire sauce
6 fl oz dark beer
3 28-oz cans crushed tomatoes
1 15-oz can black beans, rinsed and drained
1 15-oz can pinto beans, rinsed and drained
1 15-oz can red kidney beans, rinsed and drained
1 sweet potato, peeled and cubed

1. Combine spice mix ingredients in a small bowl, set aside. Heat oil in large pot or Dutch oven over medium heat. Add meat and cook until browned. Add onion, peppers, celery, and garlic and sauté for 3–5 minutes until tender, season with salt. Stir in broth, Worcestershire, beer, and crushed tomatoes. Add spice mix and stir well to combine; stir in beans and sweet potato. Bring to a simmer and cook uncovered for 25 minutes or until potatoes are tender, stirring occasionally.

Quinoa is a high-protein grain that everyone will love.

Extra prep:

- Make a large batch of chili for Wednesday night
- Cook quinoa for Tuesday

LEFTOVER TIP: Make a quick bean salad side dish with canned beans, diced bell pepper, vinaigrette dressing, and cooked quinoa.

Calories: 530
Total Fat: 14g
Saturated Fat: 1g
Carbohydrate: 76g
Protein: 30g
Sodium: 1473mg
Cholesterol: 35mg
Fiber: 18g

NUTRIENT INTAKE:

Carbs 55%

Protein 22%

Fat 23%

NUTRITION FOR THE DAY

Calories: 1544
Total Fat: 47.5g
Saturated Fat: 7.5g
Carbohydrate: 208g
Protein: 79g
Sodium: 2400mg
Cholesterol: 54mg
Fiber: 35g

NUTRIENT INTAKE:

Carbs 53%

Protein 20%

Fat 27%

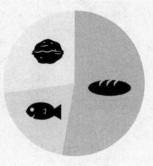

BREAKFAST

▶ **Maple Walnut Oatmeal**

MAKES 4 SERVINGS

You make this recipe with skim milk—it makes the oatmeal creamy and boosts the protein and calcium content.

2 cups rolled oats
4 cups skim milk
4 tablespoons maple syrup
4 tablespoons chopped walnuts

Walnuts are packed with omega-3 fats and the antioxidant, vitamin E.

Ground cinnamon (optional)

1. Combine oats and milk in a medium saucepan. Bring to a simmer (do not boil). Reduce heat and cook for 6 to 8 minutes or until oats are tender and the milk has been absorbed. Divide oatmeal into 4 bowls and top each serving with 1 tablespoon of syrup and walnuts; sprinkle with cinnamon if desired.

*Quick Tip: Make a double batch of oatmeal for Wednesday morning—just reheat in the microwave.

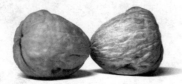

Calories: 333
Total Fat: 8g
Saturated Fat: 1g
Carbohydrate: 54g
Protein: 14g
Sodium: 105mg
Cholesterol: 5mg
Fiber: 4.5g

NUTRIENT INTAKE:

Carbs 62%
Protein 17%
Fat 21%

LUNCH

▶ **Turkey & Avocado Pita:** 3 oz low sodium turkey breast, 3 slices of avocado, baby spinach, sliced tomato, and 1 tablespoon low fat Ranch dressing in 1 whole wheat pita

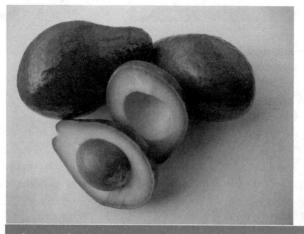

Avocado is loaded with heart-healthy unsaturated fats.

► **1 cup grapes**

Calories: 396
Total Fat: 9.5g
Saturated Fat: 1g
Carbohydrate: 55g
Protein: 36g
Sodium: 968mg
Cholesterol: 30mg
Fiber: 8g

NUTRIENT INTAKE:

Carbs 54%
Protein 25%
Fat 21%

SNACK

► **¼ cup hummus**
► **6 whole grain crackers**

Calories: 213
Total Fat: 9.5g
Saturated Fat: 1g
Carbohydrate: 27g
Protein: 7g
Sodium: 392mg
Cholesterol: 0mg
Fiber: 6g

NUTRIENT INTAKE:

Carbs 48%
Protein 13%
Fat 39%

▸ Veggie Quesadillas

SERVES: 4 (2 pieces per person)

Nonstick cooking spray
4 whole wheat tortillas
2 cups finely shredded Mexican blend cheese, divided
4 cups thinly sliced vegetables (recommendations: red onion, bell pepper, roasted red pepper, zucchini, tomato, baby spinach)
Salsa

1. Spray a nonstick pan with cooking spray and place over medium heat. Place tortilla in the pan and top with a 1 cup of cheese in an even layer, then 2 cups of vegetables. Allow to cook for 1–2 minutes to let cheese begin to melt. Top with another tortilla and gently flip over to cook on the other side. Cook until both sides are golden brown and cheese is melted. Repeat with remaining tortillas and vegetables. Cut each tortilla into 4 pieces and serve topped with salsa.

   Tip: To turn the quesadilla over, flip it onto a clean plate and slide back into the pan (uncooked side down).

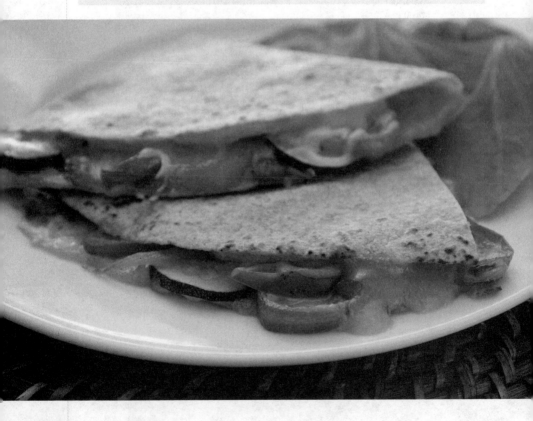

Double Duty Option:

- serve veggies and cheese rolled in the tortilla with some cooked brown rice for a veggie burrito

▶ **1 cup sliced cucumber topped with 1 tablespoon balsamic vinaigrette**

Calories: 464
Total Fat: 26g
Saturated Fat: 8g
Carbohydrate: 38g
Protein: 20g
Sodium: 860mg
Cholesterol: 38mg
Fiber: 4g

NUTRIENT INTAKE:

Carbs 33%
Protein 17%
Fat 50%

NUTRITION FOR THE DAY

Calories: 1506
Total Fat: 53g
Saturated Fat: 12g
Carbohydrate: 173g
Protein: 67g
Sodium: 2326mg
Cholesterol: 73mg
Fiber: 23g

NUTRIENT INTAKE:

Carbs 48%

Protein 22%

Fat 30%

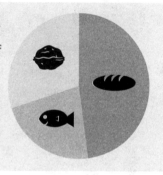

TUESDAY

BREAKFAST

▸ **Egg Sandwich:** 1 egg + 1 egg white (any style) on a whole wheat English muffin with 1 slice of low fat cheese and sliced tomato

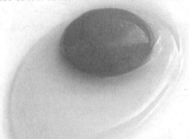

Whole wheat English muffins are great for breakfast or portion-controlled sandwiches. About 130 calories per serving.

▸ **6 fl oz orange juice**

Calories: 365
Total Fat: 8.5g
Saturated Fat: 3g
Carbohydrate: 49g
Protein: 26g
Sodium: 724mg
Cholesterol: 217mg
Fiber: 5g

NUTRIENT INTAKE:

Carbs 53%

Protein 26%

Fat 21%

LUNCH

Double Duty Option:
▸ **Peanut Butter & Jam (see Week 1)**

OR

▸ **Two slices whole wheat bread topped with 2 tablespoons almond butter and thinly sliced apple**

Almond butter is a nice change from peanut butter and just as good for you.

▸ **8 fl oz skim milk**

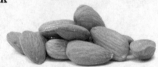

Calories: 471
Total Fat: 21.5g
Saturated Fat: 2g
Carbohydrate: 52g
Protein: 22g
Sodium: 544mg
Cholesterol: 5mg
Fiber: 10g

NUTRIENT INTAKE:

Carbs 42%
Protein 18%
Fat 40%

SNACK

▶ **6 oz nonfat fruit yogurt**

Calories: 130
Total Fat: 0g
Saturated Fat: 0g
Carbohydrate: 26g
Protein: 6g
Sodium: 105mg
Cholesterol: 0mg
Fiber: 2 g

NUTRIENT INTAKE:

Carbs 81%
Protein 19%
Fat 0%

DINNER

▶ **4 oz grilled pork tenderloin**

▶ **Quinoa Salad with Olives and Cucumber**

MAKES 6 CUPS

3 cups cooked quinoa
1 cup diced red bell pepper
1 cup pitted black olives, sliced
1 cup diced cucumber
3 scallions, finely chopped
2 tablespoons chopped fresh parsley
2 tablespoons extra virgin olive oil
Freshly squeezed lemon juice to taste
½ cup crumbled low fat feta cheese
¼ teaspoon kosher salt
¼ teaspoon black pepper to taste

1. In a large bowl combine quinoa, bell pepper, olives, cucumber, scallion, and parsley—toss to combine. Add oil, lemon juice, feta, and season with salt and pepper to taste. Toss and serve chilled or at room temperature.

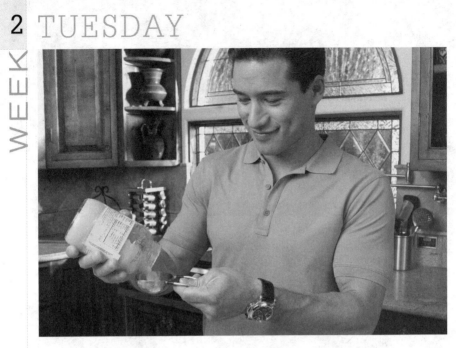

Calories: 525
Total Fat: 23g
Saturated Fat: 6g
Carbohydrate: 36g
Protein: 44g
Sodium: 475mg
Cholesterol: 123mg
Fiber: 4g

NUTRIENT INTAKE:

Carbs 27%

Protein 33%

Fat 40%

NUTRITION FOR THE DAY

Calories: 1492
Total Fat: 53g
Saturated Fat: 12g
Carbohydrate: 163g
Protein: 96g
Sodium: 1848mg
Cholesterol: 346mg
Fiber: 21g

NUTRIENT INTAKE:

Carbs 45%

Protein 30%

Fat 25%

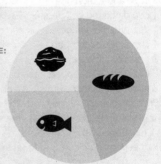

BREAKFAST

▶ **Maple Walnut Oatmeal** (see recipe on page 102)

Double Duty Option:

- top oatmeal with sliced banana and swirl in a teaspoon of peanut butter

Calories: 333
Total Fat: 8g
Saturated Fat: 1g
Carbohydrate: 54g
Protein: 14g
Sodium: 105mg
Cholesterol: 5mg
Fiber: 4.5g

NUTRIENT INTAKE:

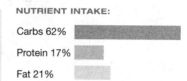

Carbs 62%
Protein 17%
Fat 21%

LUNCH

▶ **Chef's Salad:** 3 cups mixed greens topped with 2 oz grilled chicken or turkey breast, 1 oz Swiss cheese, 1 hard-boiled egg, any vegetables, and 2 tablespoons low fat Ranch dressing

Double Duty Option:

- tuck the salad ingredients into a whole wheat tortilla for a handheld lunch

Calories: 481
Total Fat: 21g
Saturated Fat: 8g
Carbohydrate: 11g
Protein: 52g
Sodium: 600mg
Cholesterol: 342mg
Fiber: 4g

NUTRIENT INTAKE:

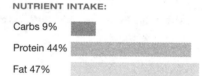

Carbs 9%
Protein 44%
Fat 47%

SNACK

▶ **1 apple**
▶ **1 tablespoon peanut or almond butter**

Calories: 235
Total Fat: 10g
Saturated Fat: 1g
Carbohydrate: 13g
Protein: 4g
Sodium: 73mg
Cholesterol: 0mg
Fiber: 7g

NUTRIENT INTAKE:

Carbs 48%
Protein 6%
Fat 46%

DINNER

► **Leftover Spicy Turkey Chili (from Sunday night)**
► **2 cups mixed greens**
► **2 tablespoons balsamic vinaigrette**

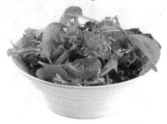

Calories: 420
Total Fat: 11g
Saturated Fat: 1g
Carbohydrate: 54g
Protein: 27g
Sodium: 1300mg
Cholesterol: 35mg
Fiber: 16g

NUTRIENT INTAKE:

Carbs 50%

Protein 25%

Fat 25%

DESSERT

► **Angel Food Cake with 60-Second Blueberry Sauce**
SERVES 8

1 cup fresh blueberries
2 teaspoons sugar
1 tablespoon freshly squeezed lemon juice
1 store-bought plain angel food cake

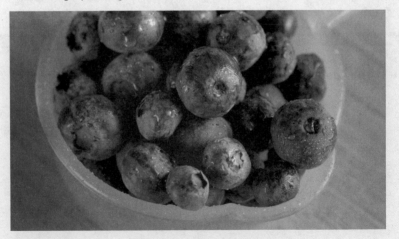

> Angel food cake—take some help from the store and get one already made; the main ingredient is egg whites, so it's light, airy, and fat free.

1. In a small bowl combine blueberries, sugar, and lemon juice. Microwave on high heat for 45 seconds. Allow sauce to cool for 5 minutes and serve over sliced angel food cake.

Calories: 139
Total Fat: 0.5g
Saturated Fat: 0g
Carbohydrate: 32g
Protein: 3g
Sodium: 319mg
Cholesterol: 0mg
Fiber: 1.5g

NUTRIENT INTAKE:

Carbs 89%

Protein 8%

Fat 3%

NUTRITION FOR THE DAY

Calories: 1547
Total Fat: 54g
Saturated Fat: 12g
Carbohydrate: 173g
Protein: 99g
Sodium: 2313mg
Cholesterol: 382mg
Fiber: 30g

NUTRIENT INTAKE:

Carbs 45%

Protein 25%

Fat 30%

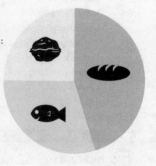

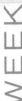
BREAKFAST

▸ 1½ cups whole grain cereal
▸ 1 cup skim milk
▸ ½ cup blueberries

Calories: 324
Total Fat: 2g
Saturated Fat: 0.5g
Carbohydrate: 67g
Protein: 15g
Sodium: 400mg
Cholesterol: 5mg
Fiber: 12g

NUTRIENT INTAKE:

Carbs 78%
Protein 17%
Fat 5%

LUNCH

▸ Leftover Quinoa Salad with Olives and Cucumber (from Wednesday)
▸ 1 apple

Calories: 385
Total Fat: 16g
Saturated Fat: 4g
Carbohydrate: 55g
Protein: 10g
Sodium: 403mg
Cholesterol: 17mg
Fiber: 7g

NUTRIENT INTAKE:

Carbs 55%
Protein 9%
Fat 36%

SNACK

▸ ¼ cup hummus
▸ 6 whole grain crackers

Calories: 213
Total Fat: 9.5g
Saturated Fat: 1g
Carbohydrate: 27g
Protein: 7g
Sodium: 392mg
Cholesterol: 0mg
Fiber: 6g

NUTRIENT INTAKE:

Carbs 48%
Protein 13%
Fat 38%

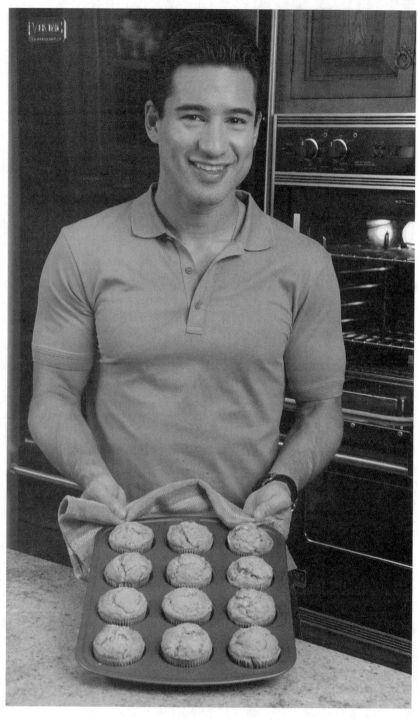

DINNER

- ► 1 cup cooked brown rice
- ► 1½ cups broccoli roasted with 1 teaspoon of sesame or canola oil

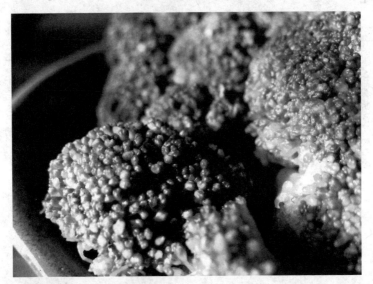

► **Orange-Glazed Salmon**

1 pound wild salmon, skin removed, cut into 4 pieces
¼ teaspoon kosher salt
¼ teaspoon black pepper
2 tablespoons reduced sodium soy sauce
2 tablespoons agave nectar
2 teaspoons freshly grated orange zest

Use the citrus peel to get orange zest; that's where all the flavor is.

1. Preheat oven to 400 degrees F. Place salmon on a baking sheet lined with parchment paper. Season with salt and pepper and place in oven to bake for 10 minutes. To make the glaze, combine soy sauce, agave, and orange zest—mix well. Remove salmon from oven, brush with glaze, return to oven, and bake for an additional 10 minutes or until cooked through.

LEFTOVER TIP: Mix leftover salmon with a few teaspoons of mayo, Greek yogurt, and chopped celery and serve on whole wheat bread with slices of fresh tomato.

Calories: 495
Total Fat: 15.5g
Saturated Fat: 2.5g
Carbohydrate: 59g
Protein: 31g
Sodium: 245mg
Cholesterol: 84mg
Fiber: 4g

NUTRIENT INTAKE:

Carbs 47%

Protein 25%

Fat 28%

NUTRITION FOR THE DAY

Calories: 1418
Total Fat: 44g
Saturated Fat: 8g
Carbohydrate: 212g
Protein: 63g
Sodium: 1610mg
Cholesterol: 106mg
Fiber: 30g

NUTRIENT INTAKE:

Carbs 55%

Protein 23%

Fat 22%

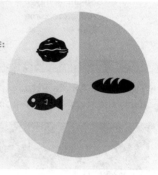

FRIDAY

BREAKFAST

▶ **1 cup nonfat Greek yogurt topped with ¾ cup blueberries and 3 tablespoons slivered almonds**

Calories: 286
Total Fat: 11g
Saturated Fat: 1g
Carbohydrate: 24g
Protein: 25g
Sodium: 86mg
Cholesterol: 0mg
Fiber: 6g

NUTRIENT INTAKE:

Carbs 36%
Protein 33%
Fat 31%

LUNCH

▶ **Turkey & Apple Pita:** 3 oz low sodium turkey breast, 1 slice low fat cheese, thinly sliced apple, mustard, and baby spinach in a whole wheat pita

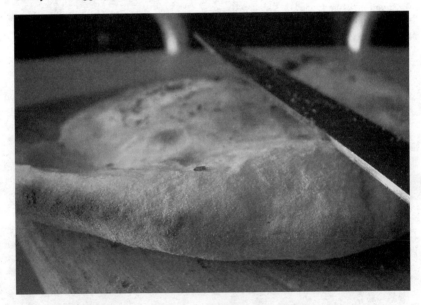

Calories: 396
Total Fat: 9.5g
Saturated Fat: 1g
Carbohydrate: 55g
Protein: 36g
Sodium: 968mg
Cholesterol: 30mg
Fiber: 8g

NUTRIENT INTAKE:

Carbs 54%
Protein 25%
Fat 21%

SNACK

▶ **6 oz nonfat fruit yogurt**

Calories: 130
Total Fat: 0g
Saturated Fat: 0g
Carbohydrate: 26g
Protein: 6g
Sodium: 105mg
Cholesterol: 0mg
Fiber: 2 g

NUTRIENT INTAKE:

Carbs 81%
Protein 19%
Fat 0%

DINNER: MAKE YOUR OWN "TAKEOUT"

▶ **Burgers & Fries**
SERVES: 4

Fries:
4 medium potatoes, scrubbed well and unpeeled
1 tablespoon canola oil
Kosher salt and black pepper

Burgers:
1 pound ground beef (90% lean)
2 tablespoons Dijon mustard
¼ cup finely chopped onion

4 whole wheat hamburger rolls
Lettuce, sliced tomato, sliced red onion, ketchup, mustard

1. To prepare fries, preheat oven to 425 degrees F. Slice potatoes into ½-inch thick fries and transfer to a baking sheet. Drizzle with oil and season with ¼ teaspoon salt and ¼ teaspoon black pepper. Bake for 30 minutes*, turning once, until golden brown. (*Cooking time may vary depending on how thin or thick fries were cut.)
2. In a large bowl, combine ground beef, mustard, ¼ teaspoon salt, and ¼ teaspoon pepper—mix gently and shape into 4 burgers. Heat grill, grill pan, or nonstick skillet over medium heat. Cook to desired doneness and serve on wheat buns with toppings.

Calories: 598
Total Fat: 19g
Saturated Fat: 7g
Carbohydrate: 70g
Protein: 38g
Sodium: 1051mg
Cholesterol: 80mg
Fiber: 8 g

NUTRIENT INTAKE:

Carbs 47%
Protein 25%
Fat 28%

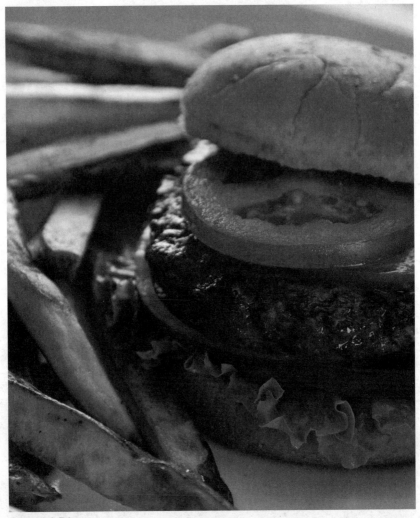

Burgers & Fries

NUTRITION FOR THE DAY

Calories: 1447
Total Fat: 39g
Saturated Fat: 9g
Carbohydrate: 178g
Protein: 95g
Sodium: 2211mg
Cholesterol: 110mg
Fiber: 22g

NUTRIENT INTAKE:

Carbs 49%

Protein 26%

Fat 25%

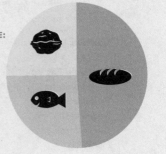

BREAKFAST

▶ **Egg Sandwich:** 1 egg + 1 egg white (any style) on a whole wheat English muffin with 1 slice of low fat cheese and sliced tomato

▶ **6 fl oz orange juice**

Calories: 365
Total Fat: 8.5g
Saturated Fat: 3g
Carbohydrate: 49g
Protein: 26g
Sodium: 724mg
Cholesterol: 217mg
Fiber: 5g

NUTRIENT INTAKE:

Carbs 53%
Protein 26%
Fat 21%

LUNCH

▶ **Cranberry Chicken Salad:** 3 cups mixed greens topped with 2 oz grilled chicken breast, 1 oz Swiss cheese, 2 tablespoons dried cranberries, any vegetables, and 2 tablespoons low fat Ranch dressing

Calories: 453
Total Fat: 19g
Saturated Fat: 7g
Carbohydrate: 23g
Protein: 46g
Sodium: 542mg
Cholesterol: 130mg
Fiber: 5g

NUTRIENT INTAKE:

Carbs 21%
Protein 41%
Fat 38%

SNACK

▶ **1 cup diced pineapple**

Calories: 74
Total Fat: 0g
Saturated Fat: 0g
Carbohydrate: 20g
Protein: 1g
Sodium: 0mg
Cholesterol: 0mg
Fiber: 2g

NUTRIENT INTAKE:

Carbs 94%
Protein 4%
Fat 2%

DINNER

▶ **Flatbreads:** 1 whole wheat pita topped with 3 oz cooked chicken breast (from a rotisserie chicken), ¼ cup shredded cheddar cheese, and sliced poblano peppers; bake until cheese is melted

Double Duty Option:

- mix up the toppings with sliced tomato and scallions

Calories: 435
Total Fat: 14g
Saturated Fat: 6g
Carbohydrate: 40g
Protein: 34g
Sodium: 596mg
Cholesterol: 102mg
Fiber: 6g

NUTRIENT INTAKE:

Carbs 36%
Protein 36%
Fat 28%

DESSERT

▶ Strawberry Frozen Yogurt

MAKES 6 1/2-CUP SERVINGS

If strawberries aren't in season, you can use frozen (unsweetened) ones or make this recipe with any seasonal fruit.

2 cups sliced strawberries
½ cup sugar
1½ cups reduced fat (2%) Greek yogurt
½ cup low fat plain yogurt

1. In a small saucepan, combine strawberries and sugar over medium heat. Bring to a simmer and cook for 15 minutes until thickened—set aside to cool completely. In a large bowl, whisk yogurts and transfer to an ice cream maker. Mix according to the manufacturer's suggestions, until thick and frosty. Add strawberry mixture to the machine and mix until well combined. Enjoy immediately or transfer to a freezer-safe container and allow to harden for one hour.

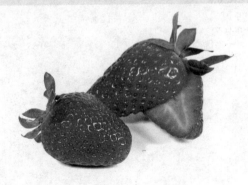

Double Duty Option:

- top with 2 tablespoons chocolate chips or crushed graham crackers

Calories: 218
Total Fat: 8g
Saturated Fat: 4.5g
Carbohydrate: 36g
Protein: 5g
Sodium: 36mg
Cholesterol: 8mg
Fiber: 2g

NUTRIENT INTAKE:

Carbs 61%

Protein 9%

Fat 30%

NUTRITION FOR THE DAY

Calories: 1546
Total Fat: 49g
Saturated Fat: 20.5g
Carbohydrate: 167g
Protein: 117g
Sodium: 1898mg
Cholesterol: 457mg
Fiber: 20g

NUTRIENT INTAKE:

Carbs 45%

Protein 30%

Fat 25%

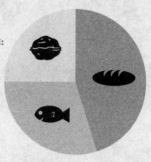

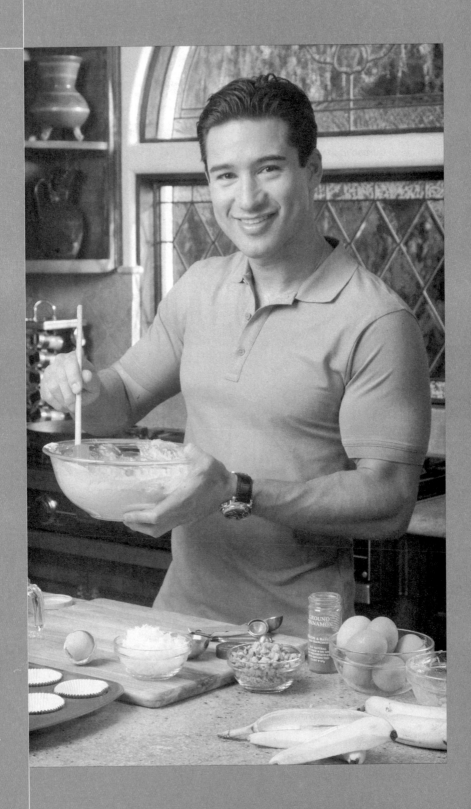

GROCERY LIST

▶ **Produce**

- ☐ Bananas: 15
- ☐ Pears: 16
- ☐ Strawberries: 3 quarts
- ☐ Melons: 2 large
- ☐ Grapes: ½ pound
- ☐ Celery: 1 bunch
- ☐ Carrots: 2
- ☐ Parsley: 1 bunch
- ☐ Cilantro: 1 bunch
- ☐ Basil: 1 bunch
- ☐ Lettuce (mixed greens or a combination of romaine and green leaf lettuces): 4 heads
- ☐ Baby spinach: 1 bag
- ☐ Spinach: 1 bunch
- ☐ Cucumbers: 3
- ☐ Tomatoes (or cherry tomatoes): 1 package cherry tomatoes or 3 tomatoes
- ☐ Garlic: 1 head
- ☐ Sweet potatoes: 4 small
- ☐ Broccoli: 1 bunch
- ☐ Onions: 5
- ☐ Scallions: 1 bunch
- ☐ Bell pepper: 1
- ☐ Lemons: 1

- ☐ Limes: 2
- ☐ Avocados: 2
- ☐ Orange juice: 3 half-gallon containers

▶ **Dairy & Eggs**

- ☐ Eggs: 3 dozen
- ☐ Skim milk: 1 half-gallon container
- ☐ Low fat chocolate milk: 2 half-gallon containers
- ☐ Low fat buttermilk: 1 pint
- ☐ Nonfat Greek yogurt: 3 large tubs
- ☐ Nonfat fruit yogurt: 4 6-ounce containers
- ☐ Shredded Mexican blend cheese: 1 package
- ☐ Feta cheese: 2 ounces
- ☐ Crumbled blue cheese: ¼ pound
- ☐ Low fat American, cheddar, or Swiss cheese (for omelet): 4 slices
- ☐ Grated Parmesan cheese

▶ **Bakery**

- ☐ Whole wheat pita: 4
- ☐ Whole wheat bread: 2 loaves
- ☐ Whole wheat English muffins: 12

☐ Whole wheat flour tortilla: 10

☐ Whole wheat hamburger rolls: 4

▶ Meat & Deli and Seafood

☐ Chicken breast (boneless, skinless): 1¾ pounds

☐ Rotisserie chicken: 2

☐ Low sodium turkey breast: ¾ pound

☐ Boneless pork chops: 4 5-ounce chops

☐ Flank steak: 1¾ pounds

☐ Ground turkey breast (or premade burgers): 1 pound

☐ Ground turkey breast: 1 pound additional (for turkey meatballs)

▶ Frozen

☐ Peas: 1 small package

☐ Vanilla ice cream: 1 pint

▶ Grocery & Pantry Items

☐ Whole grain cereal: 1 box

☐ Granola: 1 package

☐ Whole wheat pretzels: 1 bag

☐ Rolled oats: 1 canister

☐ Raw almonds

☐ Dry-roasted peanuts

☐ Dried cherries

☐ Tortilla chips: 1 bag

☐ Brown rice

☐ Whole grain pasta (such as Barilla PLUS): 1 pound

☐ Reduced sodium soy sauce

☐ Rice vinegar

☐ Balsamic vinegar

☐ Tomato paste

☐ Ketchup

☐ Mayonnaise

☐ Honey mustard

☐ Seasoned breadcrumbs: 1 small container

☐ Low sodium chicken broth

☐ Fruit spread

☐ Natural peanut butter

☐ Balsamic vinaigrette

☐ Salsa

☐ Chocolate syrup

☐ Diced tomatoes: 1 28-ounce can

☐ Canned black beans: 2 15-ounce cans

☐ Tuna, packed in water: 3 15-ounce cans

☐ Granulated sugar

☐ Whole wheat flour

☐ All-purpose flour

☐ Baking powder

☐ Baking soda

☐ Cornstarch

☐ Olive oil

☐ Canola oil

☐ Nonstick cooking spray

☐ Vanilla extract

☐ Ground cumin

☐ Cayenne pepper

☐ Chili powder

☐ Dried bay leaf

☐ Oregano

☐ Peppercorns

☐ Kosher salt

WEEK

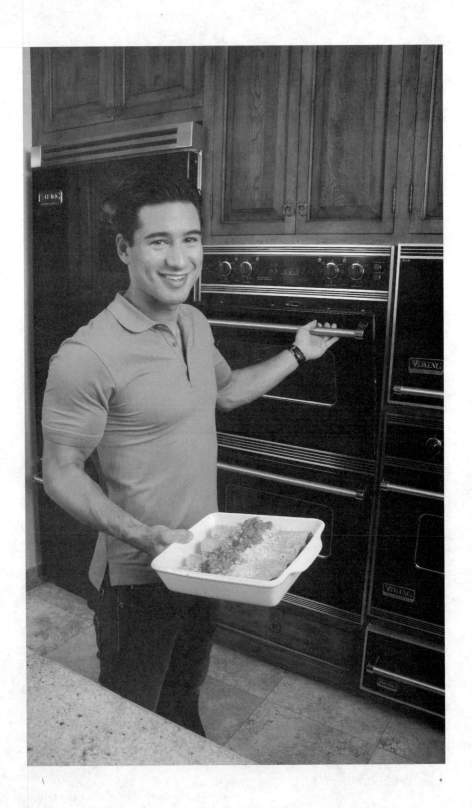

HIGHLIGHTS

Prep Day on Sunday:
- ▶ Preparing from rotisserie chicken for Chicken Enchiladas and Chicken Salad
- ▶ Using leftover parts of chicken to make homemade chicken stock that will be used throughout the week in Enchiladas, Tortilla Soup, Chicken and Broccoli
- ▶ Can replace homemade chicken stock with store-bought, low sodium version

Meatless Monday option for Week 3: Tortilla Soup—healthy fats from avocado and protein from black beans make a satisfying meatless option.

Whole grain cereal recommendations: Bran Flakes, Kashi Go Lean, or Nature's Path Multigrain Flakes

Fruits for the week: bananas, strawberries, melon, pears

Friday night's "make your own takeout" is Chinese! Much lower in calories, fat, and sodium than most of the options at the nearby Chinese take-out place.

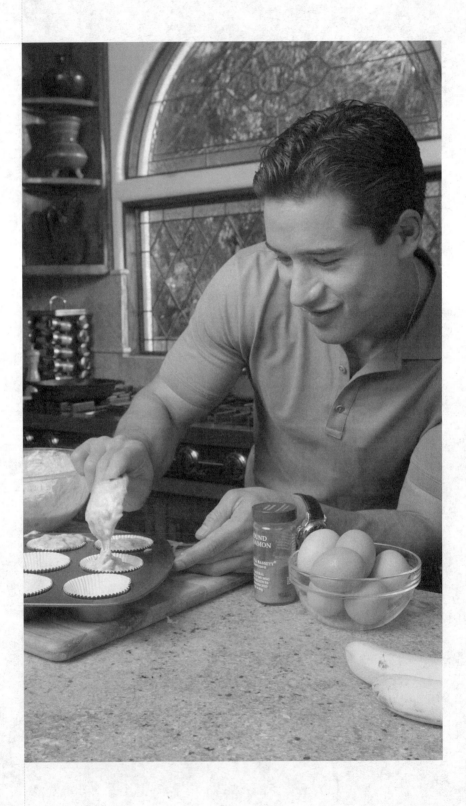

BREAKFAST

▶ **6 fl oz orange juice**

▶ **Pancakes with Strawberry Sauce**

SERVES: 4 (3 pancakes and ¼ cup strawberry sauce per serving)

2 cups of fresh or frozen strawberries
1 tablespoon sugar
2 teaspoons lemon juice

½ cup whole wheat flour
½ cup all-purpose flour
1 tablespoon sugar
1 teaspoon baking powder
½ teaspoon baking soda
Pinch salt
1 egg, lightly beaten
1 cup low fat buttermilk
¼ cup water
1 teaspoon vanilla extract
2 teaspoons canola oil
Nonstick cooking spray

1. In a small saucepan combine strawberries, sugar, and lemon juice. Cook over medium heat until berries are softened and sauce has slightly thickened—about 10 minutes.
2. In a separate bowl, sift together flours, sugar, baking power, baking soda, and salt. Add egg, buttermilk, water, vanilla, and oil; mix until just combined. Heat a nonstick pan or griddle over medium heat, spray with nonstick spray. Pour ¼ cup of batter for each pancake into pan and cook for 2 minutes per side until golden. Serve topped with strawberry sauce.

Calories: 315
Total Fat: 5g
Saturated Fat: 1g
Carbohydrate: 59g
Protein: 9g
Sodium: 399mg
Cholesterol: 55mg
Fiber: 4g

NUTRIENT INTAKE:

Carbs 74%

Protein 11%

Fat 15%

LUNCH

▶ **Greek Salad:** 3 cups mixed greens topped with 3 oz grilled chicken or turkey breast, 2 oz feta cheese, grape tomatoes, sliced cucumber, and 2 tablespoons balsamic vinaigrette

Calories: 522
Total Fat: 25g
Saturated Fat: 10.5g
Carbohydrate: 40g
Protein: 38g
Sodium: 1074mg
Cholesterol: 123mg
Fiber: 6g

NUTRIENT INTAKE:

Carbs 30%
Protein 28%
Fat 42%

SNACK

▶ **2 cups diced melon**

Calories: 106
Total Fat: 0g
Saturated Fat: 0g
Carbohydrate: 25g
Protein: 3g
Sodium: 50mg
Cholesterol: 0mg
Fiber: 3g

NUTRIENT INTAKE:

Carbs 87%
Protein 9%
Fat 4%

DINNER

▶ **Chicken Enchiladas**
SERVES: 4

1 tablespoon canola oil
½ cup chopped onion
½ cup chopped celery
1 tablespoon all-purpose flour
½ cup homemade chicken stock
½ teaspoon ground cumin
¼ teaspoon salt
Pinch cayenne pepper
4 cups shredded cooked chicken
2 cups baby spinach
4 whole wheat flour tortillas
Salsa
¾ cup shredded Mexican blend cheese
1 avocado, diced

1. Preheat oven to 350 degrees F. Spray a 9x9 square baking dish with nonstick cooking spray and set aside. Heat oil in a large skillet over medium heat. Add onions and celery and sauté for 2–3 minutes. Sprinkle with flour and cook for an additional 1 minute to allow the flour to cook. Stir in chicken stock, cumin, salt, and cayenne pepper. Add chicken and spinach and mix to combine (if mixture appears too dry, add more chicken stock). Fill each tortilla with the chicken mixture, roll up, and transfer to prepared baking dish. Top with ½ cup salsa and cheese and bake for 10–12 minutes until cheese is melted. Serve with additional salsa and diced avocado.

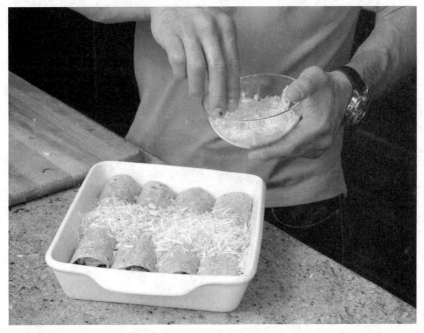

Extra Prep:

- Pick chicken from 2 rotisserie chickens for enchiladas and chicken salad recipes.
- Reserve the bones and scraps from the rotisserie chickens to make Homemade Chicken Stock.
- Can replace homemade chicken stock with store-bought, low sodium version.

▶ Homemade Chicken Stock

MAKES ABOUT 10 CUPS

Bones and scraps of 2 rotisserie chickens (2–3 pounds each)
2 carrots, cut in half
2 stalks celery, cut in half
1 onion, quartered

1 bay leaf
2 cloves garlic, whole
1½ teaspoons kosher salt
2 teaspoons peppercorns
½ bunch fresh parsley
1 dried chili-pepper (optional)
Water

1. Place chicken, vegetables, herbs, and spices in a large stock pot. Add enough water to cover contents and bring to a boil. Reduce heat and simmer for 2 hours. Strain and transfer to containers.

NUTRITION INFO PER CUP:
Calories: 86
Total Fat: 2.5g
Saturated Fat: 1g
Carbohydrate: 8g

Protein: 5g
Sodium: 335mg
Cholesterol: 7mg
Fiber: 0g

Calories: 501
Total Fat: 24g
Saturated Fat: 7g
Carbohydrate: 40g
Protein: 30g
Sodium: 811mg
Cholesterol: 68mg
Fiber: 9g

NUTRIENT INTAKE:

Carbs 33%

Protein 25%

Fat 43%

NUTRITION FOR THE DAY

Calories: 1459
Total Fat: 54g
Saturated Fat: 18.5g
Carbohydrate: 165g
Protein: 80g
Sodium: 2334mg
Cholesterol: 246mg
Fiber: 22g

NUTRIENT INTAKE:

Carbs 45%

Protein 22%

Fat 33%

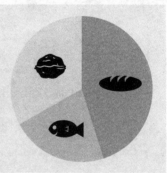

BREAKFAST

▸ **Rise & Shine Smoothie** (see recipe on page 86)

Double Duty Option:

- swap orange juice with mango or pineapple juice for a tropical flavor

Calories: 274
Total Fat: 0g
Saturated Fat: 0g
Carbohydrate: 58g
Protein: 13g
Sodium: 44mg
Cholesterol: 0mg
Fiber: 4g

NUTRIENT INTAKE:

Carbs 80%

Protein 18%

Fat 2%

LUNCH

▸ **6 oz nonfat fruit yogurt**

▸ **Chicken Salad with Fresh Herbs**

MAKES 4 SERVINGS

12 oz cooked chicken, diced or shredded
½ chopped celery stalk
2 tablespoons mayonnaise
2 tablespoons nonfat Greek yogurt
2 tablespoons finely chopped herbs (such as basil, parsley, or tarragon)
¼ teaspoon kosher salt
Freshly ground black pepper to taste
2 slices whole wheat bread

> Celery has lots of crunch for virtually no calories; celery has BIG flavor raw and even more when it's cooked.

1. Combine ingredients in a medium bowl and mix gently to combine.
2. Spread even portions in between 2 slices of whole wheat bread.

> LEFTOVER TIP: Makes enough chicken salad for half sandwiches on Thursday

Calories: 481
Total Fat: 10g
Saturated Fat: 5g
Carbohydrate: 55g
Protein: 41g
Sodium: 559mg
Cholesterol: 75mg
Fiber: 10g

NUTRIENT INTAKE:

Carbs 46%
Protein 35%
Fat 19%

SNACK

▶ Chew Cherry Trail Mix

MAKES 9 SERVINGS (⅓ cup each)

1 cup raw almonds
1 cup whole grain cereal (such as Cheerios)
½ cup dried cherries
½ cup dry-roasted peanuts

Roasting brings out the peanuts' natural flavors for no additional calories.

1. Combine ingredients in a resealable bag or airtight container. Use a ¼-cup measure as a scoop for perfect portions every time.

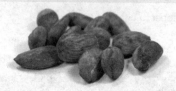

Calories: 176
Total Fat: 12g
Saturated Fat: 1g
Carbohydrate: 13g
Protein: 6g
Sodium: 24mg
Cholesterol: 0mg
Fiber: 3g

NUTRIENT INTAKE:

Carbs 28%
Protein 13%
Fat 59%

DINNER

▶ **2 cups mixed greens**
▶ **2 tablespoons balsamic vinaigrette**

► **Tortilla Soup**

MAKES 8 SERVINGS

1 tablespoon canola oil
½ cup chopped red onion
½ cup chopped celery
½ cup chopped carrot
1 bell pepper, diced (if you want more spice, use a poblano pepper)
1 teaspoon chili powder
6 cups chicken broth
15-oz can black beans, rinsed and drained
¼ cup chopped cilantro
1 avocado, diced
Tortilla chips, crushed (5 per serving)
Lime wedges (optional)

1. Heat oil in a large stock pot over medium heat. Add onion, celery, carrot, and pepper; season with chili powder and sauté for 2 minutes. Add chicken broth and black beans and cook for an additional 10 minutes. Serve soup in large bowls topped with diced avocado, tortilla chips, and a squeeze of fresh lime juice, if desired.

Extra Prep:

- While the soup is cooking, prepare 1 cup (dry) brown rice for dinner Friday night.

Calories: 521
Total Fat: 25.5g
Saturated Fat: 3g
Carbohydrate: 63g
Protein: 15g
Sodium: 1100mg
Cholesterol: 15mg
Fiber: 5g

NUTRIENT INTAKE:

Carbs 47%

Protein 11%

Fat 52%

NUTRITION FOR THE DAY

Calories: 1553
Total Fat: 48g
Saturated Fat: 6g
Carbohydrate: 188g
Protein: 75g
Sodium: 1728mg
Cholesterol: 80mg
Fiber: 28g

NUTRIENT INTAKE:

Carbs 51%

Protein 24%

Fat 26%

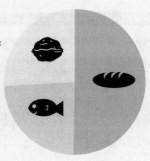

TUESDAY

BREAKFAST

- ▶ 2 eggs, scrambled with ½ cup vegetables
- ▶ 1 toasted whole wheat English muffin
- ▶ 1 pear

Calories: 395
Total Fat: 11.5g
Saturated Fat: 3.5g
Carbohydrate: 56g
Protein: 20g
Sodium: 374mg
Cholesterol: 423mg
Fiber: 7g

NUTRIENT INTAKE:

Carbs 55%
Protein 20%
Fat 25%

LUNCH

- ▶ Tuna Salad with Grapes (see recipe on page 76) on whole wheat pita

LEFTOVER TIP: Mix water-packed (drained) tuna, celery, shredded carrot, and balsamic vinaigrette with cooked whole grain pasta for an instant pasta salad.

- ▶ 1 oz whole wheat pretzels

Calories: 438
Total Fat: 9g
Saturated Fat: 1g
Carbohydrate: 56g
Protein: 39g
Sodium: 795mg
Cholesterol: 49mg
Fiber: 5g

NUTRIENT INTAKE:

Carbs 48%
Protein 34%
Fat 18%

SNACK

- ▶ 6 fl oz low fat chocolate milk

Get calcium and vitamin D for growing bones—studies have found that chocolate milk also makes a great post-workout recovery drink.

- ▶ 1 banana

Calories: 223
Total Fat: 2g
Saturated Fat: 0.5g
Carbohydrate: 25g
Protein: 9g
Sodium: 25mg
Cholesterol: 3mg
Fiber: 2g

NUTRIENT INTAKE:

Carbs 79%
Protein 12%
Fat 9%

DINNER

- ▶ 4 oz turkey burgers (get premade burgers or mix 1 pound ground turkey breast with ¼ cup finely chopped onion and 2 tablespoons mustard. Makes 4 burgers.)
- ▶ 4 whole wheat rolls
- ▶ 2 cups mixed greens topped with 1 tablespoon each balsamic vinaigrette and crumbled blue cheese

Double Duty Option:

- top burgers with blue cheese

LEFTOVER TIP: Sauté ground turkey with a combination of marinara sauce and BBQ sauce for homemade Sloppy Joes.

Calories: 442
Total Fat: 16g
Saturated Fat: 6g
Carbohydrate: 34g
Protein: 40g
Sodium: 962mg
Cholesterol: 91mg
Fiber: 5g

NUTRIENT INTAKE:

Carbs 31%
Protein 36%
Fat 33%

NUTRITION FOR THE DAY

Calories: 1498
Total Fat: 39g
Saturated Fat: 12g
Carbohydrate: 193g
Protein: 106g
Sodium: 2246mg
Cholesterol: 569mg
Fiber: 21g

NUTRIENT INTAKE:

Carbs 50%
Protein 26%
Fat 24%

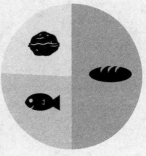

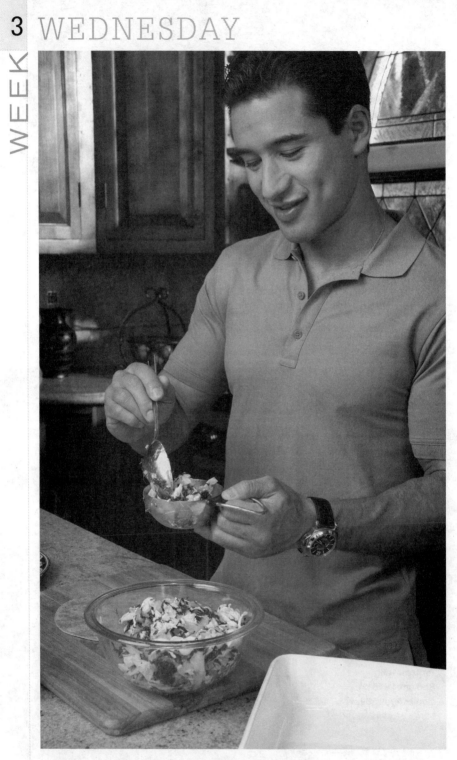

BREAKFAST

▶ **1 cup cooked oatmeal topped with ⅓ cup granola**
▶ **6 fl oz orange juice**

Calories: 459
Total Fat: 5g
Saturated Fat: 0.5g
Carbohydrate: 95g
Protein: 11g
Sodium: 366mg
Cholesterol: 0mg
Fiber: 7g

NUTRIENT INTAKE:

Carbs 81%
Protein 9%
Fat 10%

LUNCH

▶ **Turkey & Cheese Wrap:** 3 oz low sodium turkey breast, sliced tomato, lettuce, and honey mustard in a whole wheat flour tortilla

Honey mustard is a lighter alternative to mayo. Make your own with equal parts honey and spicy or Dijon mustard.

▶ **1 pear**

Calories: 318
Total Fat: 4g
Saturated Fat: 0g
Carbohydrate: 51g
Protein: 17g
Sodium: 364mg
Cholesterol: 20mg
Fiber: 7g

NUTRIENT INTAKE:

Carbs 67%
Protein 22%
Fat 11%

SNACK

▶ **Chewy Cherry Trail Mix (see recipe on page 134)**

Calories: 176
Total Fat: 12g
Saturated Fat: 1g
Carbohydrate: 13g
Protein: 6g
Sodium: 24mg
Cholesterol: 0mg
Fiber: 3g

NUTRIENT INTAKE:

Carbs 28%
Protein 13%
Fat 59%

WEDNESDAY

DINNER

► **Chili-rubbed Pork Chops:** season a 5-oz boneless pork chop with chili powder, lime juice, and a drizzle of canola oil, and grill
► **2 cups broccoli, roasted with 2 teaspoons extra virgin olive oil**

Calories: 446
Total Fat: 26g
Saturated Fat: 7g
Carbohydrate: 8g
Protein: 46g
Sodium: 126mg
Cholesterol: 120mg
Fiber: 0g

NUTRIENT INTAKE:

Carbs 7%

Protein 41%

Fat 52%

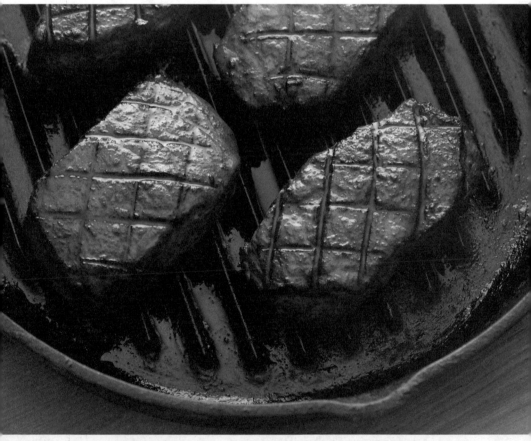

Chili-rubbed Pork Chops

DESSERT

▶ **Fruit Parfaits:** ¾ cup nonfat Greek yogurt layered in a glass with ½ cup each sliced strawberries and bananas. Top with 2 tablespoons granola.

Calories: 216
Total Fat: 1g
Saturated Fat: 0g
Carbohydrate: 36g
Protein: 18g
Sodium: 64mg
Cholesterol: 0mg
Fiber: 4g

NUTRIENT INTAKE:

Carbs 65%

Protein 32%

Fat 3%

NUTRITION FOR THE DAY

Calories: 1605
Total Fat: 48g
Saturated Fat: 8g
Carbohydrate: 202g
Protein: 98g
Sodium: 1146mg
Cholesterol: 140mg
Fiber: 22g

NUTRIENT INTAKE:

Carbs 50%

Protein 27%

Fat 23%

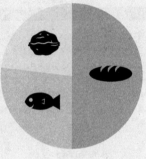

THURSDAY

BREAKFAST

- ► 2 eggs, scrambled with ½ cup vegetables
- ► 1 toasted whole wheat English muffin
- ► 1 pear

Calories: 395
Total Fat: 11.5g
Saturated Fat: 3.5g
Carbohydrate: 56g
Protein: 20g
Sodium: 374mg
Cholesterol: 423mg
Fiber: 7g

NUTRIENT INTAKE:

Carbs 55%
Protein 20%
Fat 25%

LUNCH

- ► 1 banana
- ► 1 cup leftover Tortilla Soup
- ► ½ chicken salad sandwich (from Monday)

Double Duty Option:

- ▪ serve chicken salad over mixed greens with chopped tomato

Calories: 482
Total Fat: 19.5g
Saturated Fat: 3g
Carbohydrate: 51g
Protein: 28g
Sodium: 784mg
Cholesterol: 43mg
Fiber: 10g

NUTRIENT INTAKE:

Carbs 42%
Protein 22%
Fat 36%

SNACK

- ► 6 fl oz low fat chocolate milk

Calories: 223
Total Fat: 2g
Saturated Fat: 0.5g
Carbohydrate: 25g
Protein: 9g
Sodium: 25mg
Cholesterol: 3mg
Fiber: 2g

NUTRIENT INTAKE:

Carbs 75%
Protein 11%
Fat 14%

DINNER

- ▸ 4 oz grilled flank steak
- ▸ 1 cup steamed spinach topped with 1 teaspoon olive oil and lemon juice
- ▸ 1 small baked sweet potato topped with 2 tablespoons nonfat Greek yogurt

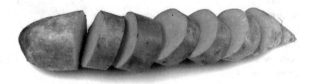

Extra Prep:

- Grill extra steak for lunch tomorrow

Double Duty Option:

- make stuffed sweet potatoes with veggies and a dollop of Greek yogurt

Calories: 431
Total Fat: 14g
Saturated Fat: 4.5g
Carbohydrate: 29g
Protein: 47g
Sodium: 328mg
Cholesterol: 61mg
Fiber: 4g

NUTRIENT INTAKE:

Carbs 27%
Protein 43%
Fat 30%

NUTRITION FOR THE DAY

Calories: 1556
Total Fat: 49g
Saturated Fat: 13g
Carbohydrate: 186g
Protein: 101g
Sodium: 1610mg
Cholesterol: 542mg
Fiber: 25g

NUTRIENT INTAKE:

Carbs 47%
Protein 25%
Fat 28%

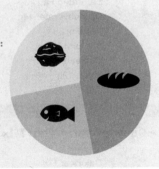

FRIDAY

BREAKFAST

- 1½ cups whole grain cereal
- 1 cup skim milk
- ½ cup sliced strawberries

Calories: 311
Total Fat: 2g
Saturated Fat: 0.5g
Carbohydrate: 67g
Protein: 15g
Sodium: 400mg
Cholesterol: 5mg
Fiber: 12g

NUTRIENT INTAKE:

Carbs 78%
Protein 17%
Fat 5%

LUNCH

- 1 pear

Double Duty Option

- **Beef Taco Wraps:** 2–3 slices cooked steak with lettuce, salsa, and shredded cheese in a whole wheat wrap

OR

- **Tex Mex Salad:** 3 cups mixed greens topped with 3 oz grilled steak, grape tomatoes, sliced cucumber, ¼ cup black beans, ¼ cup shredded cheese, 2 teaspoons olive oil, and lime juice to taste

Calories: 569
Total Fat: 28g
Saturated Fat: 10g
Carbohydrate: 44g
Protein: 36g
Sodium: 509mg
Cholesterol: 62mg
Fiber: 12g

NUTRIENT INTAKE:

Carbs 31%
Protein 25%
Fat 44%

SNACK

- **Chewy Cherry Trail Mix (see recipe on page 134)**

Calories: 176
Total Fat: 12g
Saturated Fat: 1g
Carbohydrate: 13g
Protein: 6g
Sodium: 24mg
Cholesterol: 0mg
Fiber: 3g

NUTRIENT INTAKE:

Carbs 28%
Protein 13%
Fat 59%

DINNER: MAKE YOUR OWN "TAKEOUT"

▶ Sweet and Sour Chicken & Broccoli and Fried Rice

SERVES: 4

Sweet and Sour Sauce:
½ cup chicken broth
2 tablespoons reduced sodium soy sauce

> **Make the switch** from regular soy sauce and you'll save over 400 milligrams of sodium per tablespoon.

2 tablespoons ketchup
2 tablespoons sugar
2 tablespoons rice vinegar
2 teaspoons cornstarch
1 teaspoon chili sauce (optional)
1 tablespoon canola oil

1 pound boneless, skinless chicken breast, diced
4 cups broccoli florets

Fried Rice:
1 tablespoon canola oil
½ cup diced scallion
3 cups cooked brown rice
1 egg, beaten
1 cup frozen peas, thawed
1 tablespoon reduced sodium soy sauce

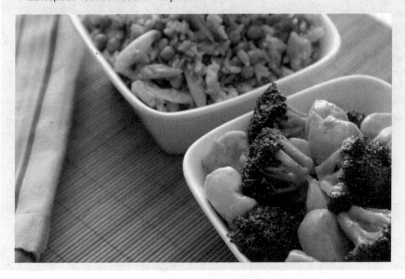

1. For the chicken and broccoli: combine the ingredients for the sweet and sour sauce, whisk well to combine and set aside. Heat oil in a large wok or skillet over high heat. Add chicken and cook for 2–3 minutes until browned. Reduce heat to medium-high, add broccoli and sauce and continue to cook, tossing frequently until chicken is cooked through and broccoli is slightly tender, 5–6 minutes more. Transfer to a large serving dish and wipe out the pan with a paper towel. For the rice, heat oil in the same wok (or skillet) over high heat; add scallion and cook for 30 seconds to infuse the oil with the onion flavor. Add rice and cook until warmed—about 1–2 minutes. Make a well in the center of the rice and add beaten egg, gently scramble egg and slowly incorporate it into the rice. Add peas and soy sauce.

LEFTOVER TIP: Dip pieces of grilled chicken in a peanut sauce made from natural peanut butter, rice vinegar, and a few dashes of soy sauce or hot sauce.

Calories: 475
Total Fat: 12g
Saturated Fat: 2g
Carbohydrate: 55g
Protein: 37g
Sodium: 528mg
Cholesterol: 120mg
Fiber: 4.5g

NUTRIENT INTAKE:

Carbs 47%

Protein 24%

Fat 29%

NUTRITION FOR THE DAY

Calories: 1524
Total Fat: 55g
Saturated Fat: 14g
Carbohydrate: 178g
Protein: 94g
Sodium: 1605mg
Cholesterol: 186mg
Fiber: 32g

NUTRIENT INTAKE:

Carbs 47%

Protein 24%

Fat 29%

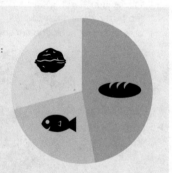

BREAKFAST

- ▸ **1 toasted whole wheat English muffin**
- ▸ **1 cup strawberries**

- ▸ **Mix-n-Match Omelet**

  A breakfast to please everyone. Choose any combination of veggies and cheese for a scrumptious morning meal.

  SERVES: 1

  Nonstick cooking spray
  1 egg + 2 egg whites
  1 tablespoon water
  Salt and pepper to taste
  ½ cup vegetables (suggestions: mushrooms, bell peppers, tomatoes, baby spinach)
  1 slice low fat cheese

  1. Heat a nonstick skillet over medium heat. Combine egg, egg whites, and water in a bowl, season with salt and pepper, and whisk well. Add vegetables to eggs. Spray skillet with nonstick spray and add egg mixture. Cook for 3–4 minutes until eggs begin to set. Using a rubber spatula, gently pull in the sides of the omelet to let the uncooked egg run to the edges of the pan. Place cheese on one side of the omelet and gently fold in half. Allow to cook for 2 minutes until cheese is melted. Slide omelet onto a plate.

Calories: 401
Total Fat: 10.5g
Saturated Fat: 3.5g
Carbohydrate: 49g
Protein: 20g
Sodium: 374mg
Cholesterol: 423mg
Fiber: 8g

NUTRIENT INTAKE:

Carbs 41%
Protein 35%
Fat 24%

LUNCH

- ▸ **Peanut Butter & Jam:** 2 slices whole wheat bread topped with 2 tablespoons peanut butter and 1 tablespoon fruit spread

Calories: 423
Total Fat: 19g
Saturated Fat: 3g
Carbohydrate: 50g
Protein: 14g
Sodium: 351mg
Cholesterol: 0mg
Fiber: 8g

NUTRIENT INTAKE:

Carbs 47%
Protein 13%
Fat 40%

SNACK

▶ **2 cups diced melon**

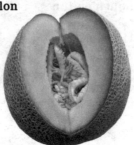

Calories: 106
Total Fat: 0g
Saturated Fat: 0g
Carbohydrate: 25g
Protein: 3g
Sodium: 50mg
Cholesterol: 0mg
Fiber: 3g

NUTRIENT INTAKE:

Carbs 87%
Protein 9%
Fat 4%

DINNER

▶ **2 cups mixed greens**
▶ **1 tablespoon balsamic vinaigrette**

▶ **Spaghetti and Meatballs**

SERVES: 4

A favorite from the original Extra Lean plan. Got any extra vegetables on hand? Toss them in the sauce!

1 tablespoon olive oil
1 cup diced onion
2 cloves garlic, minced
¼ teaspoon kosher salt
⅛ teaspoon black pepper
2 tablespoons tomato paste
28-oz can diced tomatoes
¼ cup fresh basil, chopped

1 lb ground turkey breast
¼ cup minced onion
1 clove garlic, minced
2 teaspoons dried oregano
¼ cup seasoned breadcrumbs
1 egg, lightly beaten

¼ teaspoon kosher salt
¼ teaspoon black pepper

8 oz whole grain pasta (such as Barilla PLUS)

For the sauce:
   Heat oil in a medium saucepan; add onion and garlic and cook for 7–10 minutes. Season with salt and pepper. Add tomato paste, diced tomatoes, and basil. Reduce heat and simmer for 20 minutes.

For the meatballs:
1. Preheat oven to 375 degrees F. In a bowl combine turkey, onion, garlic, oregano, breadcrumbs, egg, salt, and pepper. Mix gently to combine and form into meatballs. Transfer to a baking sheet lined with parchment paper and bake for 30 minutes. When meatballs are cooked, add them to pot with sauce.
2. Cook pasta according to package directions, drain. Serve pasta with meatballs and sauce.

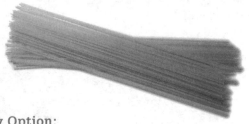

Double Duty Option:
- make a "meatball sub" by serving the meatballs in a whole wheat hamburger bun with a sprinkle of part-skim mozzarella cheese

Calories: 480
Total Fat: 6.5g
Saturated Fat: 1g
Carbohydrate: 66g
Protein: 42g
Sodium: 949mg
Cholesterol: 124mg
Fiber: 3g

NUTRIENT INTAKE:

Carbs 54%
Protein 34%
Fat 12%

DESSERT

▶ Ice Cream Sundaes

½ cup vanilla ice cream topped with 1 tablespoon chopped walnuts or almonds

Light and low fat ice creams are often loaded with preservatives. Get the real stuff instead but keep the portions modest.

Double Duty Option:

- in addition to the nuts, top with 2 tablespoons chocolate syrup—OR leftover strawberry sauce from Sunday morning breakfast

Calories: 242
Total Fat: 13.5g
Saturated Fat: 3g
Carbohydrate: 28g
Protein: 4g
Sodium: 49mg
Cholesterol: 35mg
Fiber: 1g

NUTRIENT INTAKE:

Carbs 45%
Protein 6%
Fat 49%

NUTRITION FOR THE DAY

Calories: 1540
Total Fat: 47g
Saturated Fat: 13g
Carbohydrate: 200g
Protein: 88g
Sodium: 1765mg
Cholesterol: 380mg
Fiber: 21g

NUTRIENT INTAKE:

Carbs 51%
Protein 22%
Fat 27%

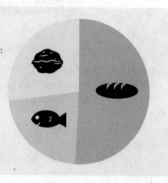

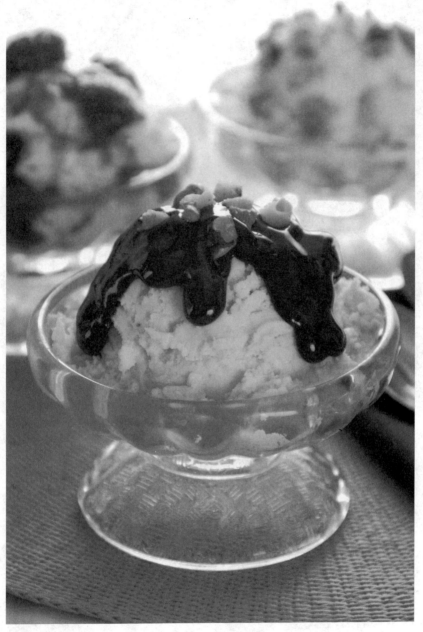

Ice Cream Sundaes

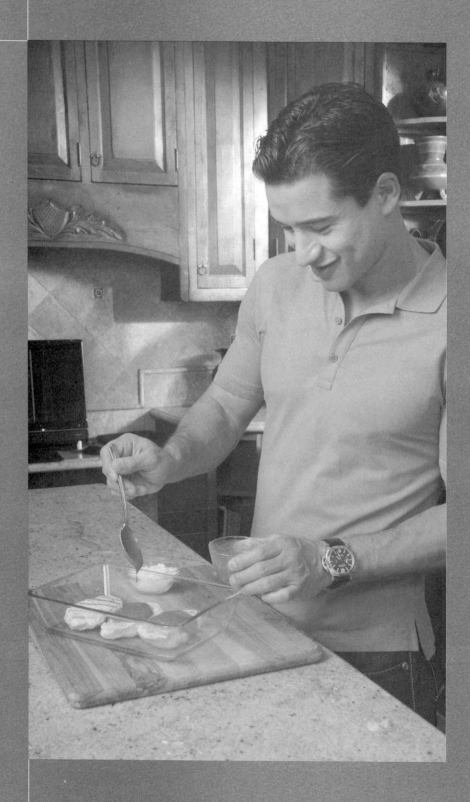

GROCERY LIST

▶ **Produce**

☐ Apples: 20

☐ Bananas: 8

☐ Raspberries: 1 pint

☐ Pineapples: 2

☐ Orange: 1

☐ Grapes: 4 pounds

☐ Chives: 1 bunch

☐ Lettuce (mixed greens or a combination of romaine and green leaf lettuces): 4 heads

☐ Spinach: 2 heads

☐ Cucumbers: 3

☐ Baby carrots: 1 bag

☐ Carrots: 1 bunch

☐ White mushrooms: 1 small package

☐ Tomatoes (or cherry tomatoes): 9 medium or 3 containers cherry tomatoes

☐ Garlic: 1 head

☐ Yukon Gold potatoes: 4 small

☐ Sweet potatoes: 4 medium

☐ Broccoli: 1 bunch

☐ Onions: 3

☐ Scallions: 1 bunch

☐ Bell peppers: 3 peppers (at least 1 red)

☐ Green beans: 1 pound

☐ Lemons: 1

☐ Lime: 1

☐ Avocados: 2

▶ **Dairy & Eggs**

☐ Eggs: 1½ dozen

☐ Skim milk: 1 gallon

☐ Low fat (1%) milk: 1 pint

☐ Heavy cream: 1 pint

☐ Whipped cream: 1 can

☐ Swiss cheese: 4 ounces

☐ Nonfat Greek yogurt: 3 large tubs

☐ Reduced fat cream cheese (or Neufchatel): 1 container

☐ Shredded cheddar cheese: 1 package

☐ String cheese: 1 package of 8 sticks

☐ Shredded provolone cheese: 1 package

☐ Crumbled feta cheese: ½ pound

☐ Shredded mozzarella cheese: 1 package

☐ Grated Parmesan cheese: 1 container

☐ Unsalted butter: 1 stick

☐ Nonfat chocolate pudding: 1 large tub or 4 snack-size cups

▶ Bakery

- ☐ Whole grain bread: 1 loaf
- ☐ Whole wheat pita: 4
- ☐ Whole wheat bread: 1 loaf
- ☐ Whole wheat English muffins: 4

▶ Meat & Deli and Seafood

- ☐ Chicken breast (boneless, skinless): 4¼ pounds
- ☐ Ground turkey breast: 1 pound
- ☐ Low sodium turkey breast: ¾ pound
- ☐ Turkey bacon: 4 slices
- ☐ Beef tenderloin or London broil: 1¼ pounds
- ☐ Wild salmon: 1 pound
- ☐ Hummus: 2 large tubs

▶ Grocery & Pantry Items

- ☐ Whole grain cereal (such as Cheerios): 1 box
- ☐ Granola: 1 package
- ☐ Graham crackers: 1 box
- ☐ Corn taco shells: 8
- ☐ Rolled oats: 1 canister
- ☐ Raw almonds
- ☐ Chopped walnuts
- ☐ Sweetened shredded coconut: 1 package
- ☐ Raisins: 1 small container
- ☐ Brown rice
- ☐ Whole grain elbow macaroni (like whole wheat or Barilla PLUS): 1 pound

- ☐ Penne (or bow-tie) pasta: 1 16-ounce box
- ☐ Reduced sodium soy sauce
- ☐ Balsamic vinegar
- ☐ Ketchup
- ☐ Hot sauce
- ☐ Panko breadcrumbs: 1 small package
- ☐ Natural peanut butter
- ☐ Apple butter
- ☐ Balsamic vinaigrette
- ☐ Low fat Ranch dressing
- ☐ Tomato sauce
- ☐ Salsa
- ☐ Maple syrup
- ☐ Unsweetened applesauce
- ☐ Agave nectar
- ☐ Garbanzo beans: 1 15-ounce can
- ☐ Black olives: 2 cans
- ☐ Mandarin oranges: 1 large can (water- or juice-packed)
- ☐ Granulated sugar
- ☐ Confectioners' sugar
- ☐ Dark brown sugar
- ☐ Whole wheat pastry flour
- ☐ All-purpose flour
- ☐ Baking powder
- ☐ Baking soda
- ☐ Olive oil
- ☐ Canola oil
- ☐ Toasted sesame oil
- ☐ Nonstick cooking spray
- ☐ Vanilla extract

- ☐ Ground nutmeg
- ☐ Ground cinnamon
- ☐ Chili powder
- ☐ Celery salt

- ☐ Ground cumin
- ☐ Kosher salt
- ☐ Black pepper

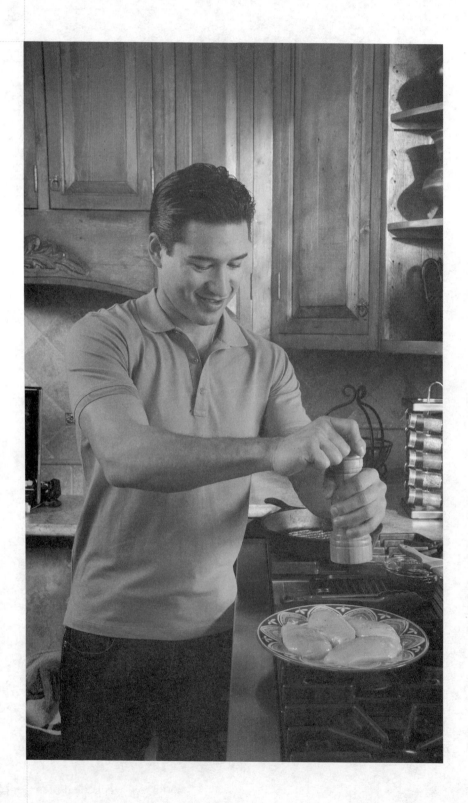

HIGHLIGHTS

Prep Day on Sunday:
- ▶ Rainbow Pasta Salad recipe will be lunch for 2 days this week
- ▶ Banana-Coconut Muffins will be for breakfast 2 days—freeze leftovers
- ▶ Grill or bake chicken breast for Wednesday night dinner

Meatless Monday option for Week 4: Spinach and Red Pepper Frittata—breakfast food for dinner is always fun! Loading the eggs up with veggies makes it healthy and satisfying.

Whole grain cereal recommendations: Bran Flakes, Kashi Go Lean, or Nature's Path Multigrain Flakes

Fruits for the week: apples, raspberries, bananas, pineapple, grapes, mandarin oranges

Friday night's "make your own takeout" is Mexican! Who doesn't love a taco? Each member of the family can pick and choose their favorite toppings—this makes a healthy meal—none of the greasy, cheesy overload you might get at the drive-through.

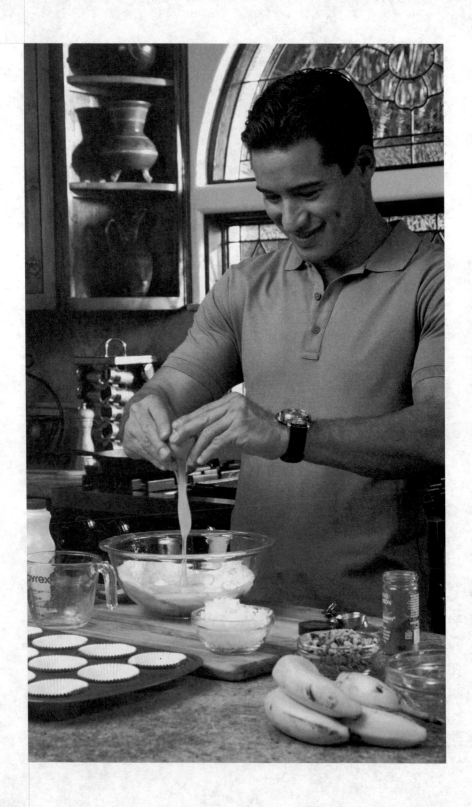

BREAKFAST

- ► 1½ cups whole grain cereal
- ► 1 cup skim milk
- ► ½ cup raspberries

Each cup of raspberries has more than 30 percent of your daily fiber needs.

Calories: 327
Total Fat: 2g
Saturated Fat: 0.5g
Carbohydrate: 67g
Protein: 15g
Sodium: 400mg
Cholesterol: 5mg
Fiber: 13g

NUTRIENT INTAKE:
Carbs 77%
Protein 17%
Fat 6%

LUNCH

- ► **Sesame Chicken Salad:** 3 cups mixed greens topped with 4 oz cooked chicken breast, sliced cucumber, ¼ cup black olives, ½ cup mandarin oranges, 2 teaspoons sesame oil, and lime juice to taste

Sesame oil is a highly flavorful oil, a little goes a long way.

Calories: 444
Total Fat: 20g
Saturated Fat: 3g
Carbohydrate: 27g
Protein: 37g
Sodium: 232mg
Cholesterol: 96mg
Fiber: 3g

NUTRIENT INTAKE:
Carbs 25%
Protein 34%
Fat 41%

SNACK

- ► 1 cup grapes

Calories: 110
Total Fat: 0g
Saturated Fat: 0g
Carbohydrate: 29g
Protein: 1g
Sodium: 3mg
Cholesterol: 0mg
Fiber: 1.5g

NUTRIENT INTAKE:
Carbs 94%
Protein 4%
Fat 2%

DINNER

▶ Bacon & Cheddar Macaroni Casserole

SERVES: 4

¾ pound whole grain elbow macaroni (like whole wheat or Barilla PLUS)
1 tablespoon unsalted butter
½ cup diced onion
½ teaspoon kosher salt
½ teaspoon black pepper
1 tablespoon all-purpose flour
1 cup low fat (1%) milk
2 tablespoons reduced fat cream cheese (Neufchatel cheese)
¾ cup shredded cheddar cheese
Pinch ground nutmeg
4 slices cooked turkey bacon, finely chopped
1 cup chopped tomato
Nonstick cooking spray

1 slice whole wheat bread
2 tablespoons grated Parmesan cheese
1 teaspoon olive oil
1 clove garlic

1. Preheat oven to 350 degrees F. Cook pasta according to package directions. While pasta is cooking, melt butter in a large saucepan. Add onion, salt, and pepper, and sauté for 5 minutes. Sprinkle flour over onions and cook, stirring constantly for 1 minute. Whisk in milk and simmer until thickened. Stir in cream cheese, cheddar, and nutmeg and cook until cheese is melted—turn off heat. Add drained pasta to cheese mixture along with turkey bacon and tomatoes and mix well. Transfer to a baking dish sprayed with nonstick cooking spray. For the topping, place bread, cheese, oil, and garlic in a food processor fitted with a steel blade; pulse until bread is in fine crumbs. Sprinkle breadcrumbs over pasta and bake for 10 minutes until golden.

LEFTOVER TIP: Make BLTs with leftover turkey bacon with lots of fresh lettuce and tomato on a whole wheat English muffin.

Calories: 575
Total Fat: 19.5g
Saturated Fat: 8.5g
Carbohydrate: 72g
Protein: 28g
Sodium: 636mg
Cholesterol: 55mg
Fiber: 8g

NUTRIENT INTAKE:

Carbs 50%

Protein 19%

Fat 31%

NUTRITION FOR THE DAY

Calories: 1445
Total Fat: 42g
Saturated Fat: 12.5g
Carbohydrate: 196g
Protein: 81g
Sodium: 1442mg
Cholesterol: 157mg
Fiber: 27g

NUTRIENT INTAKE:

Carbs 53%

Protein 22%

Fat 25%

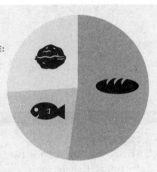

MONDAY

BREAKFAST

► Maple Walnut Oatmeal (see recipe on page 102)
► 1 apple

Quick Tip:
- make a double batch of oatmeal for Wednesday morning

Calories: 438
Total Fat: 8g
Saturated Fat: 1g
Carbohydrate: 81g
Protein: 16g
Sodium: 106mg
Cholesterol: 5mg
Fiber: 7.5g

NUTRIENT INTAKE:

Carbs 70%
Protein 14%
Fat 16%

LUNCH

► 1 cup grapes
► **Turkey & Avocado Pita:** 3 oz low sodium turkey breast, 3 slices of avocado, baby spinach, sliced tomato, and 1 tablespoon low fat Ranch dressing in 1 whole wheat pita

Double Duty Option:
- turn this into a salad and save almost 200 calories

Calories: 396
Total Fat: 9.5g
Saturated Fat: 1g
Carbohydrate: 55g
Protein: 36g
Sodium: 968mg
Cholesterol: 30mg
Fiber: 8g

NUTRIENT INTAKE:

Carbs 54%
Protein 25%
Fat 21%

SNACK

▶ 1 string cheese

String cheese is made with part-skim mozzarella, a great handheld way to get protein and calcium.

▶ 15 almonds

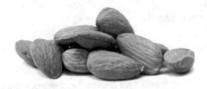

Calories: 184
Total Fat: 15g
Saturated Fat: 4.5g
Carbohydrate: 5g
Protein: 11g
Sodium: 220mg
Cholesterol: 20mg
Fiber: 2g

NUTRIENT INTAKE:

Carbs 9%

Protein 22%

Fat 69%

DINNER

▶ 2 slices whole wheat bread, toasted
▶ 1 cup cherry tomatoes, halved, topped with
▶ 1 tablespoon balsamic vinaigrette

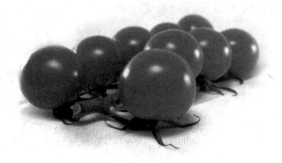

▶ Spinach & Red Pepper Frittata

SERVES: 4

8 large eggs
2 tablespoons water
¼ teaspoon kosher salt
⅛ teaspoon black pepper
1 cup diced red bell pepper
1 cup cooked spinach
½ cup shredded provolone cheese
1 tablespoon olive oil
¼ cup grated Parmesan cheese

1. Preheat broiler. In a large bowl, beat eggs and water; season with salt and pepper. Mix in bell pepper, spinach, and provolone cheese. Heat an oven-safe skillet over medium heat, add oil and swirl to coat the bottom of the pan. Pour in egg mixture and gently stir with a rubber spatula until eggs are almost completely set. Sprinkle with Parmesan cheese and transfer to the oven to brown the top. Watch carefully to make sure it does not burn! Allow to cool slightly; slice and serve.

Calories: 544
Total Fat: 30g
Saturated Fat: 8g
Carbohydrate: 41g
Protein: 29g
Sodium: 1050mg
Cholesterol: 439mg
Fiber: 11.5g

NUTRIENT INTAKE:

Carbs 30%

Protein 21%

Fat 49%

NUTRITION FOR THE DAY

Calories: 1562
Total Fat: 63g
Saturated Fat: 15g
Carbohydrate: 181g
Protein: 81g
Sodium: 2305mg
Cholesterol: 494mg
Fiber: 29g

NUTRIENT INTAKE:

Carbs 45%

Protein 25%

Fat 30%

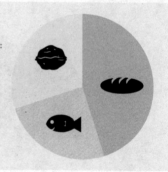

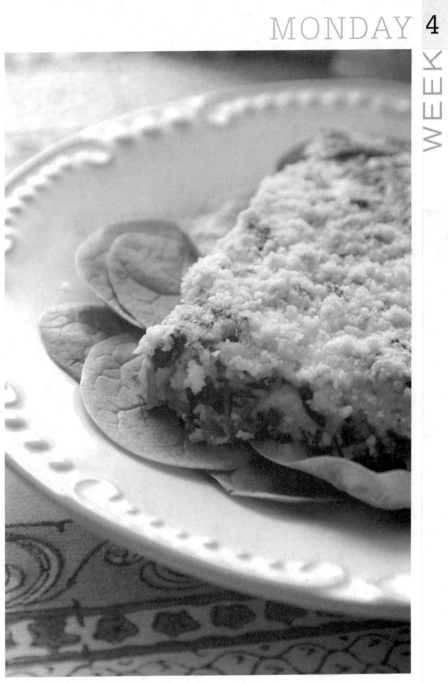

Spinach & Red Pepper Frittata

▶ **1 apple**

▶ **Banana-Coconut Muffins**

MAKES 12 MUFFINS

Freeze leftover muffins in a plastic bag—microwave for 15–30 seconds to reheat.

¾ cup whole wheat pastry flour

Whole wheat pastry flour is softer than regular whole wheat flour, which makes it perfect for baking.

¾ cup all-purpose flour
¼ cup sugar
½ teaspoon baking powder
1 teaspoon baking soda
¼ teaspoon ground cinnamon
½ teaspoon salt

1 cup mashed banana (about 2 bananas)
¼ cup unsweetened applesauce
¼ cup canola oil
½ cup low fat milk
1 large egg
1 teaspoon vanilla extract
¾ cup chopped walnuts
¼ cup sweetened shredded coconut

1. Preheat oven to 375 degrees F. Line a muffin pan with paper liners. In a large bowl combine flours, sugar, baking powder, baking soda, cinnamon, and salt. Make a well in the center of the dry ingredients and add banana, applesauce, canola oil, milk, egg, and vanilla; mix gently to combine. Fold in walnuts and coconut. Using a ⅓-cup measure, scoop batter into muffin pans and bake for 20–25 minutes until puffed and golden.

Calories: 272
Total Fat: 11g
Saturated Fat: 1.5g
Carbohydrate: 42g
Protein: 4g
Sodium: 107mg
Cholesterol: 18mg
Fiber: 5.5g

NUTRIENT INTAKE:

Carbs 59%

Protein 6%

Fat 35%

LUNCH

▶ **Greek Salad:** 3 cups mixed greens topped with 3 oz grilled chicken or turkey breast, 2 oz feta cheese, grape tomatoes, sliced cucumber, and 2 tablespoons balsamic vinaigrette

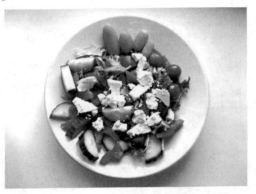

Calories: 522
Total Fat: 25g
Saturated Fat: 10.5g
Carbohydrate: 40g
Protein: 38g
Sodium: 1074mg
Cholesterol: 123mg
Fiber: 6g

NUTRIENT INTAKE:

Carbs 30%
Protein 28%
Fat 42%

SNACK

▶ **10 baby carrots**

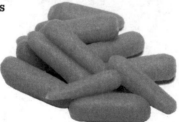

▶ **½ cup hummus**

Calories: 175
Total Fat: 6g
Saturated Fat: 0g
Carbohydrate: 24g
Protein: 5g
Sodium: 538mg
Cholesterol: 0mg
Fiber: 6g

NUTRIENT INTAKE:

Carbs 57%
Protein 11%
Fat 32%

DINNER

- ▸ Orange-Glazed Salmon (see recipe on page 114)
- ▸ 1 cup cooked brown rice
- ▸ 1½ cups broccoli roasted with 1 teaspoon of sesame or canola oil

Double Duty Option:

- ▪ serve with cooked quinoa instead of rice—it cooks in half the time

Calories: 495
Total Fat: 15.5g
Saturated Fat: 2.5g
Carbohydrate: 59g
Protein: 31g
Sodium: 245mg
Cholesterol: 84mg
Fiber: 4g

NUTRIENT INTAKE:

Carbs 47%

Protein 25%

Fat 28%

NUTRITION FOR THE DAY

Calories: 1465
Total Fat: 57g
Saturated Fat: 14g
Carbohydrate: 166g
Protein: 78g
Sodium: 1959mg
Cholesterol: 225mg
Fiber: 20.5g

NUTRIENT INTAKE:

Carbs 44%

Protein 25%

Fat 31%

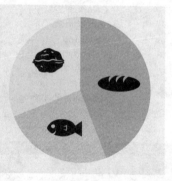

BREAKFAST

▶ **Maple Walnut Oatmeal (see recipe on page 102)**
▶ **1 apple**

Double Duty Option:

- top oatmeal with raspberries and swirl in a teaspoon of almond butter

Calories: 438
Total Fat: 8g
Saturated Fat: 1g
Carbohydrate: 81g
Protein: 16g
Sodium: 106mg
Cholesterol: 5mg
Fiber: 7.5g

NUTRIENT INTAKE:

Carbs 65%

Protein 15%

Fat 20%

LUNCH

▶ **Rainbow Pasta Salad**

MAKES 8 SERVINGS

1 pound penne or bow-tie pasta
1 medium red bell pepper, diced
1 cup diced cucumber
1 cup sliced black olives
½ cup shredded carrots
15-oz can garbanzo beans, rinsed and drained
½ cup crumbled feta cheese

Crumbled feta cheese has a salty flavor and creamy texture and is naturally lower in fat than many other cheeses.

¼ cup balsamic vinaigrette salad dressing

1. Cook pasta according to package directions. Toss cooked pasta with remaining ingredients. Serve chilled or at room temperature.

Calories: 356
Total Fat: 9.5g
Saturated Fat: 2g
Carbohydrate: 55g
Protein: 11g
Sodium: 368mg
Cholesterol: 8mg
Fiber: 4.5g

NUTRIENT INTAKE:

Carbs 62%

Protein 13%

Fat 25%

SNACK

▶ 1 apple
▶ 1 tablespoon peanut butter

Calories: 177
Total Fat: 9g
Saturated Fat: 1.5g
Carbohydrate: 22g
Protein: 4g
Sodium: 16mg
Cholesterol: 0mg
Fiber: 5g

NUTRIENT INTAKE:

Carbs 48%
Protein 6%
Fat 46%

DINNER

▶ **Baked Chicken Parmesan*:** 4 oz grilled chicken breast topped with ¼ cup tomato sauce and ¼ cup shredded mozzarella cheese; bake at 350 degrees until cheese is melted.

*make extra for tomorrow's lunch

▶ 1 slice whole grain bread
▶ 2 cups mixed greens
▶ 2 tablespoons balsamic vinaigrette

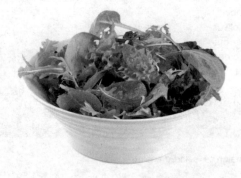

Calories: 432
Total Fat: 21g
Saturated Fat: 6g
Carbohydrate: 17g
Protein: 44g
Sodium: 879mg
Cholesterol: 111mg
Fiber: 1.5g

NUTRIENT INTAKE:

Carbs 16%
Protein 40%
Fat 44%

DESSERT

► Ice Box Cake Parfaits

MAKES 4 SERVINGS

A decadent but guilt-free dessert. Use real whipped cream, but watch those portions—it has 25 calories per tablespoon!

2 cups nonfat chocolate pudding
8 sheets graham crackers, crushed
2 bananas, sliced
4 tablespoons whipped cream

1. Prepare each serving in a small bowl or glass. Layer ½ cup pudding, crushed graham crackers, bananas, and top with whipped cream.

Calories: 239
Total Fat: 5g
Saturated Fat: 2g
Carbohydrate: 47g
Protein: 5g
Sodium: 280mg
Cholesterol: 12mg
Fiber: 3g

NUTRIENT INTAKE:

Carbs 75%
Protein 7%
Fat 18%

NUTRITION FOR THE DAY

Calories: 1533
Total Fat: 53g
Saturated Fat: 12g
Carbohydrate: 195g
Protein: 77g
Sodium: 1706mg
Cholesterol: 137mg
Fiber: 17g

NUTRIENT INTAKE:

Carbs 50%
Protein 22%
Fat 28%

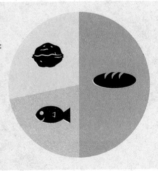

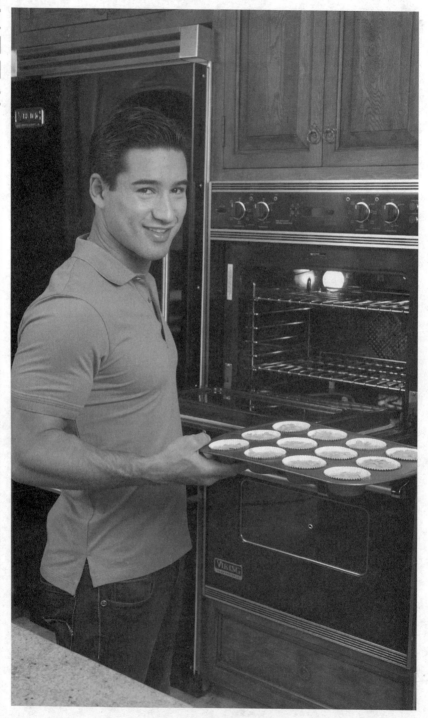

BREAKFAST

▶ **Banana-Coconut Muffin (leftovers from Tuesday)**
▶ **1 apple**

Calories: 272
Total Fat: 11g
Saturated Fat: 1.5g
Carbohydrate: 42g
Protein: 4g
Sodium: 107mg
Cholesterol: 18mg
Fiber: 5.5g

NUTRIENT INTAKE:

Carbs 59%
Protein 6%
Fat 35%

LUNCH

▶ **Chicken Parm Sandwiches:** 1 piece leftover baked chicken Parmesan, 1 slice whole wheat bread. Top with a handful of baby spinach or mixed greens
▶ **1 cup grapes**

Double Duty Option:

- use the leftover for dinner instead with 1-cup portions of cooked whole wheat pasta

Calories: 471
Total Fat: 13g
Saturated Fat: 5g
Carbohydrate: 41g
Protein: 47g
Sodium: 653mg
Cholesterol: 111mg
Fiber: 5.5g

NUTRIENT INTAKE:

Carbs 35%
Protein 40%
Fat 25%

SNACK

▶ **1 string cheese**
▶ **15 almonds**

Calories: 184
Total Fat: 15g
Saturated Fat: 4.5g
Carbohydrate: 5g
Protein: 11g
Sodium: 220mg
Cholesterol: 20mg
Fiber: 2g

NUTRIENT INTAKE:

Carbs 9%
Protein 22%
Fat 69%

THURSDAY

DINNER

- ► 5 oz grilled steak (beef tenderloin or London broil)
- ► 1 cup steamed spinach topped with 1 teaspoon olive oil and lemon juice
- ► 1 small baked Yukon Gold potato topped with 2 tablespoons nonfat Greek yogurt

Calories: 578
Total Fat: 13g
Saturated Fat: 3.5g
Carbohydrate: 56g
Protein: 61g
Sodium: 648mg
Cholesterol: 102mg
Fiber: 10g

NUTRIENT INTAKE:

Carbs 38%
Protein 42%
Fat 20%

NUTRITION FOR THE DAY

Calories: 1505
Total Fat: 52g
Saturated Fat: 14g
Carbohydrate: 143g
Protein: 123g
Sodium: 1622mg
Cholesterol: 251mg
Fiber: 23g

NUTRIENT INTAKE:

Carbs 40%
Protein 32%
Fat 31%

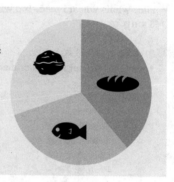

BREAKFAST

▶ **1 cup nonfat Greek yogurt topped with ¾ cup pineapple and ⅓ cup granola**

> **Granola** has a healthy crunch from grains and nuts and natural sweetness from fruit. Check labels and get one with minimal amounts of added sugar.

Calories: 413
Total Fat: 6g
Saturated Fat: 0g
Carbohydrate: 66g
Protein: 28g
Sodium: 92mg
Cholesterol: 0mg
Fiber: 7g

NUTRIENT INTAKE:

Carbs 61%
Protein 26%
Fat 13%

LUNCH

▶ **Rainbow Pasta Salad (leftovers from Wednesday or make a new batch)**

Double Duty Option:

▪ add some diced turkey, lean ham, or chicken breast for some more protein

Calories: 356
Total Fat: 9.5g
Saturated Fat: 2g
Carbohydrate: 55g
Protein: 11g
Sodium: 368mg
Cholesterol: 8mg
Fiber: 4.5g

NUTRIENT INTAKE:

Carbs 62%
Protein 13%
Fat 25%

SNACK

▶ **10 baby carrots**
▶ **½ cup hummus**

Calories: 175
Total Fat: 6g
Saturated Fat: 0g
Carbohydrate: 24g
Protein: 5g
Sodium: 538mg
Cholesterol: 0mg
Fiber: 6g

NUTRIENT INTAKE:

Carbs 57%
Protein 11%
Fat 32%

▶ Taco Night

SERVES: 4

1 tablespoon canola oil
½ cup chopped onion
½ cup diced bell pepper
1 pound ground turkey breast
1 teaspoon chili powder
1 teaspoon celery salt
½ teaspoon ground cumin

Crunchy corn taco shells (2 per person)
Hot sauce (optional)

1 cup of each of the following toppings:
     Shredded lettuce
     Chopped tomato
     Sliced black olives
     Shredded cheese
     Nonfat Greek yogurt
     Diced avocado
     Sliced red onion or chopped scallions
     Salsa

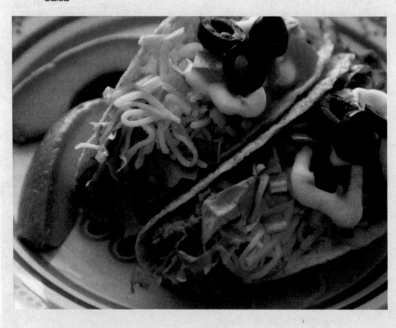

1. To prepare taco filling, heat oil in a large skillet over medium heat. Add onions and peppers and sauté for 2–3 minutes. Add turkey and spices and cook, breaking up with a spatula until turkey is completely cooked. Serve in taco shells with desired toppings.

Calories: 532
Total Fat: 24g
Saturated Fat: 6g
Carbohydrate: 37g
Protein: 42g
Sodium: 520mg
Cholesterol: 90mg
Fiber: 7g

NUTRIENT INTAKE:

Carbs 27%
Protein 32%
Fat 41%

NUTRITION FOR THE DAY

Calories: 1476
Total Fat: 46g
Saturated Fat: 8g
Carbohydrate: 181g
Protein: 86g
Sodium: 1808mg
Cholesterol: 98mg
Fiber: 24g

NUTRIENT INTAKE:

Carbs 49%
Protein 23%
Fat 28%

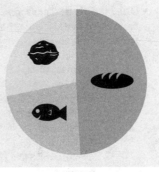

BREAKFAST

▶ 2 eggs, scrambled with ½ cup vegetables
▶ 1 toasted whole wheat English muffin
▶ 1 banana

Calories: 395
Total Fat: 11.5g
Saturated Fat: 3.5g
Carbohydrate: 56g
Protein: 20g
Sodium: 374mg
Cholesterol: 423mg
Fiber: 7g

NUTRIENT INTAKE:

Carbs 55%
Protein 20%
Fat 25%

LUNCH

▶ **Chefs' Salad:** 3 cups mixed greens topped with 2 oz grilled chicken or turkey breast, 1 oz Swiss cheese, 1 hard-boiled egg, any vegetables, and 2 tablespoons low fat Ranch dressing

Calories: 481
Total Fat: 21g
Saturated Fat: 8g
Carbohydrate: 11g
Protein: 52g
Sodium: 600mg
Cholesterol: 342mg
Fiber: 4g

NUTRIENT INTAKE:

Carbs 9%
Protein 44%
Fat 47%

SNACK

▶ 1 cup diced pineapple

Calories: 74
Total Fat: 0g
Saturated Fat: 0g
Carbohydrate: 20g
Protein: 1g
Sodium: 2 mg
Cholesterol: 0mg
Fiber: 0g

NUTRIENT INTAKE:

Carbs 94%
Protein 4%
Fat 2%

DINNER

▶ **Turkey Meatloaf with Mashed Sweet Potatoes and Roasted String Beans**

SERVES: 4

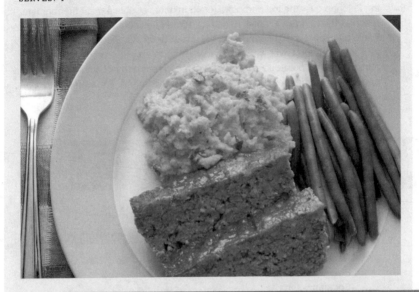

When buying ground turkey, always get ground breast meat. "Ground turkey" also contains dark meat and skin, which is higher in fat and calories.

Nonstick cooking spray
1 pound ground turkey breast
½ cup finely chopped onion
½ cup finely chopped mushrooms
1 egg, beaten
1 tablespoon balsamic vinegar
½ cup Panko breadcrumbs
Kosher salt and freshly ground black pepper
2 tablespoons ketchup, divided

4 medium sweet potatoes, peeled and diced
2 tablespoons butter
2 tablespoons nonfat Greek yogurt
Chopped chives (optional)

1 pound green beans, trimmed and steamed in the microwave for 3 minutes

1. Preheat oven to 375 degrees F. Spray a loaf pan with nonstick cooking spray. In a large bowl combine turkey, onion, mushrooms, egg, vinegar, breadcrumbs, ¼ teaspoon salt, ¼ teaspoon pepper, and 1 tablespoon ketchup. With clean hands, mix gently and just enough to combine the ingredients. Transfer the mixture to the prepared pan and gently pat to make an even layer. Spread remaining ketchup over the top and bake for 45 minutes or until a meat thermometer reaches 160 degrees F. Allow to rest for 10 minutes before slicing.
2. While meatloaf is cooking, prepare the sweet potatoes. Place diced potatoes in a large pot and cover with cool water. Bring to a boil and cook for 15–20 minutes or until potatoes are tender. Drain and return to pot; season with ½ teaspoon salt and pepper and mash with butter and yogurt. Top with fresh chives, if desired.

Use the same ingredients for Turkey Meatloaf recipe and make turkey burgers—they will cook in half the time.

Calories: 452
Total Fat: 8g
Saturated Fat: 4g
Carbohydrate: 58g
Protein: 37g
Sodium: 568mg
Cholesterol: 139mg
Fiber: 10g

NUTRIENT INTAKE:

Carbs 51%

Protein 33%

Fat 16%

DESSERT

► **Oatmeal Raisin Cookies**
This recipe makes 20 large cookies. Freeze the extras or have the kids take them to school to share with the class.

6 tablespoons softened butter
½ cup granulated sugar
½ cup dark brown sugar
1 large egg
1 teaspoon vanilla extract
1 cup rolled oats
½ cup all-purpose flour
½ cup whole wheat pastry flour
½ teaspoon baking soda
¼ teaspoon salt
¼ teaspoon cinnamon
½ cup raisins (for extra-plump raisins, soak them in hot water for 10 minutes and drain before adding to the cookie dough)

1. Preheat oven to 350 degrees F. Line a baking sheet with parchment paper and set aside. Combine butter, sugars, egg, and vanilla in the bowl of a mixer fitted with a paddle attachment. Mix on medium speed for 2 minutes, until fluffy. In a separate bowl combine oats, flours, baking soda, salt, and cinnamon. On low speed, add the dry ingredients to the mixer bowl and mix until just combined. Turn off the mixer and fold in the raisins using a spatula. Spoon large tablespoons of dough onto the baking sheet—keep them at least 2 inches apart. Bake for 13–15 minutes. Allow to cool on the baking sheet for 5 minutes and then transfer to a cooling rack to cool completely.

2. For an extra treat—make icing! Combine ¼ cup confectioners' sugar with 1 tablespoon heavy cream. Mix well and drizzle over cooled cookies.

NUTRITION PER SERVING WITHOUT THE ICING (icing adds 9 calories per serving):

Calories: 120
Total Fat: 3.5g
Saturated Fat: 0g
Carbohydrate: 21g
Protein: 2g
Sodium: 57mg
Cholesterol: 11mg
Fiber: 1.5g

NUTRIENT INTAKE:

Carbs 68%
Protein 6%
Fat 26%

NUTRITION FOR THE DAY

Calories: 1522
Total Fat: 47g
Saturated Fat: 16g
Carbohydrate: 165g
Protein: 112g
Sodium: 1604mg
Cholesterol: 614mg
Fiber: 25g

NUTRIENT INTAKE:

Carbs 43%
Protein 29%
Fat 28%

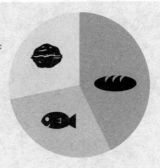

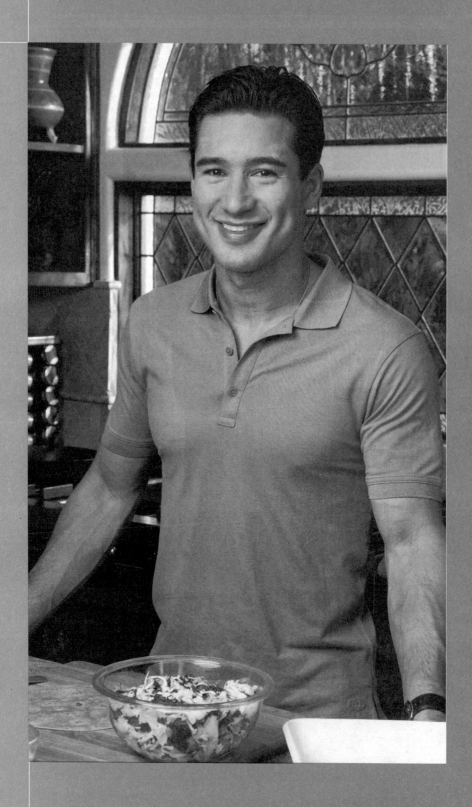

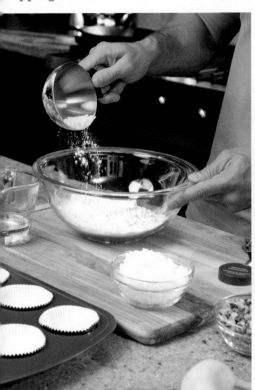
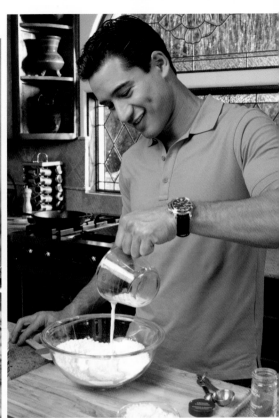
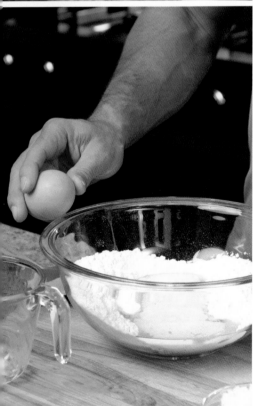
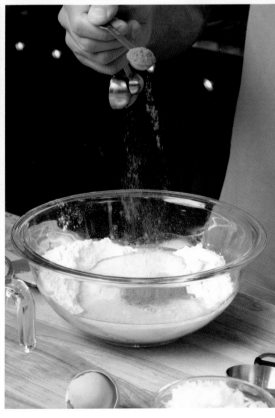

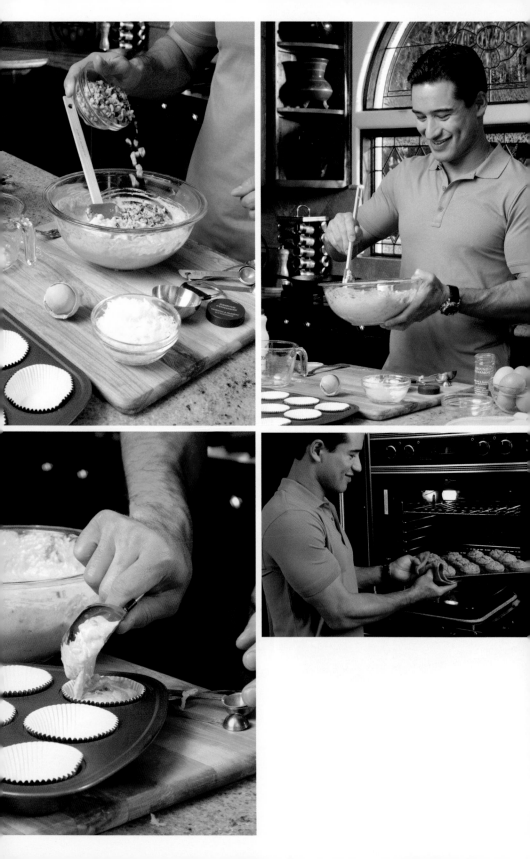

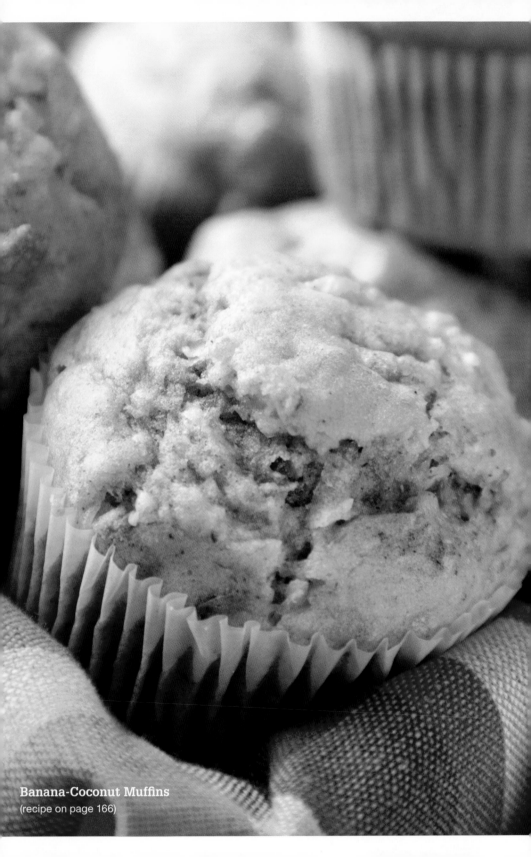

Banana-Coconut Muffins
(recipe on page 166)

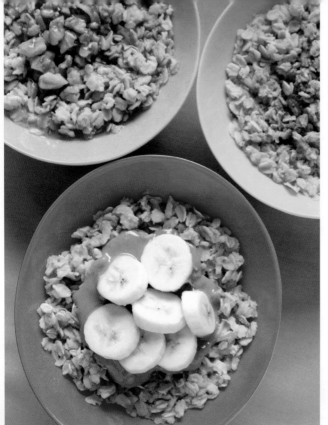

**Maple Walnut Oatmeal,
Double Duty Options**
(recipes on pages 102, 109)

**Cinnamon-Banana French
Toast** (recipe on page 69)

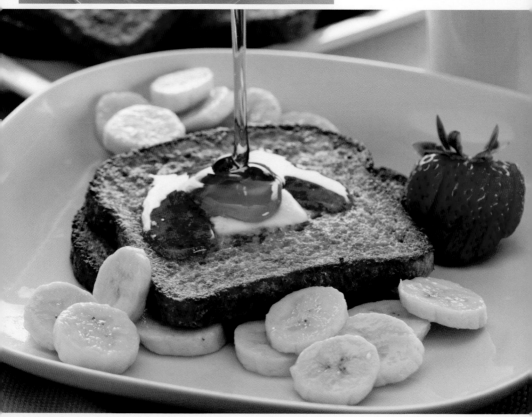

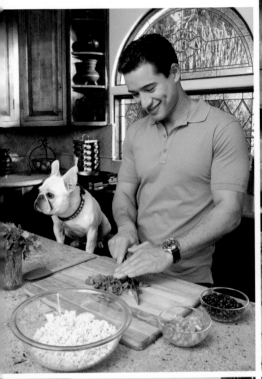
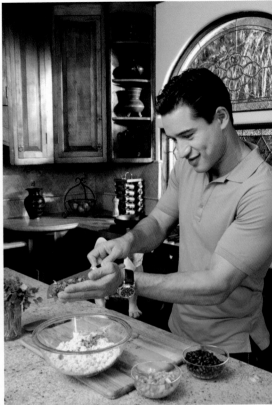
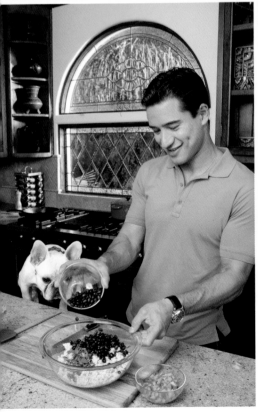
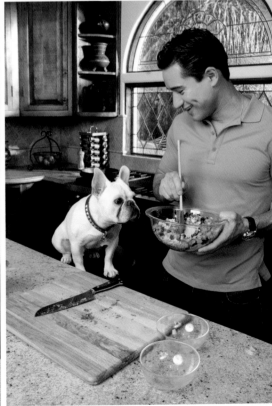

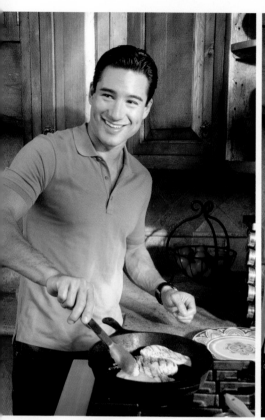
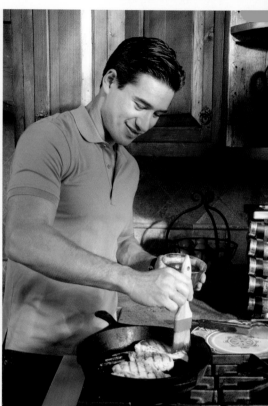
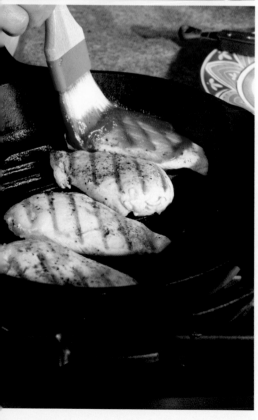

Prepping the BBQ chicken

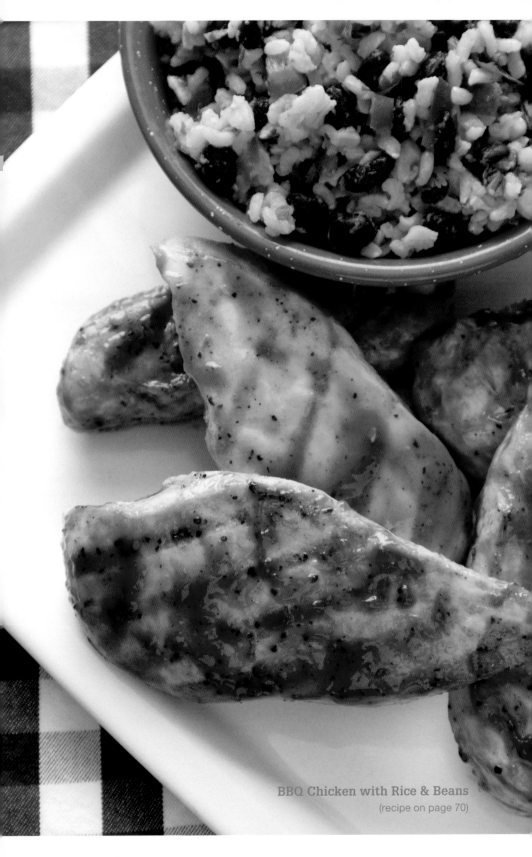

BBQ Chicken with Rice & Beans
(recipe on page 70)

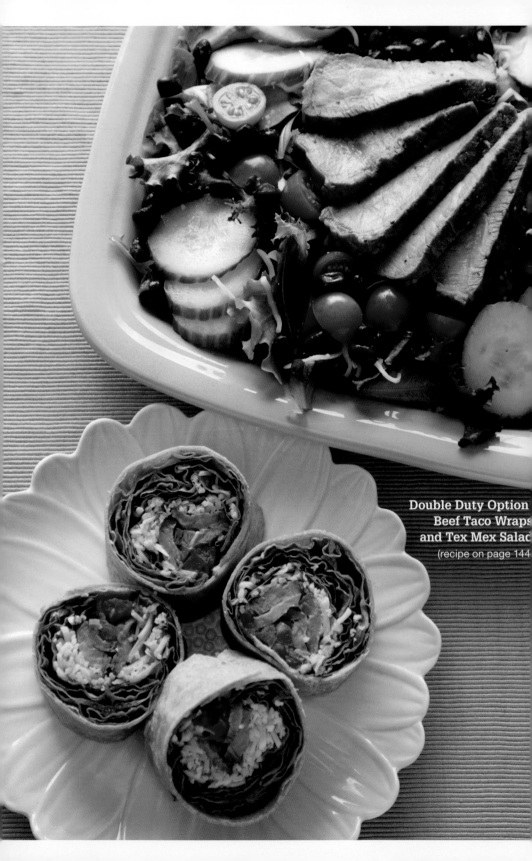

Double Duty Option
Beef Taco Wraps
and Tex Mex Salad
(recipe on page 144)

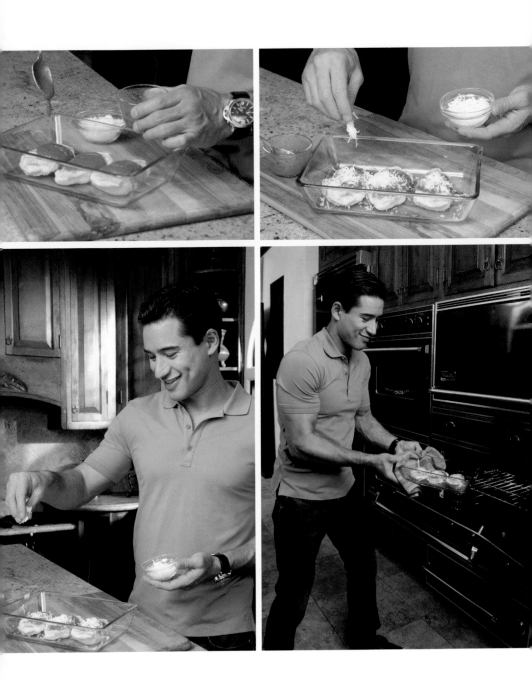

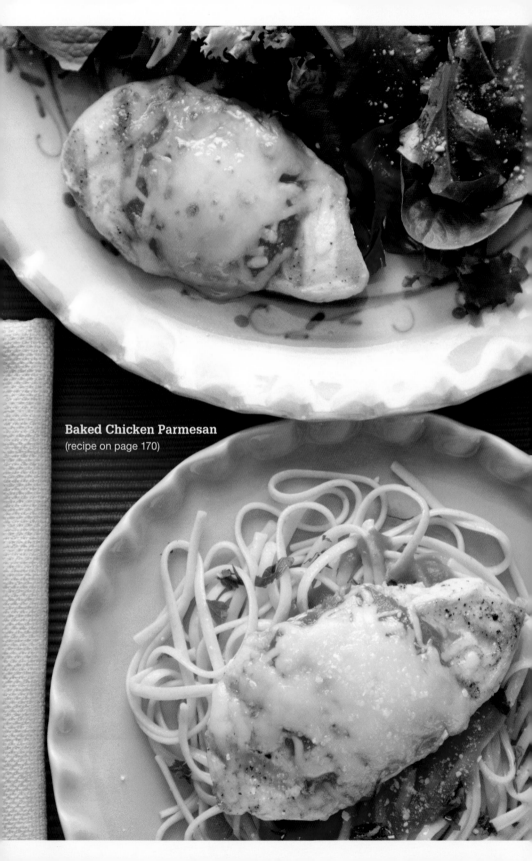

Baked Chicken Parmesan
(recipe on page 170)

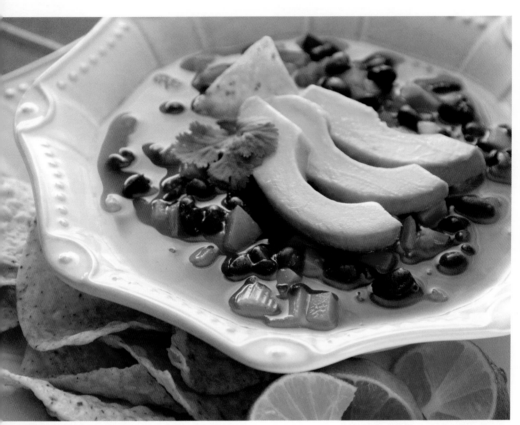

Tortilla Soup (recipe on page 135)

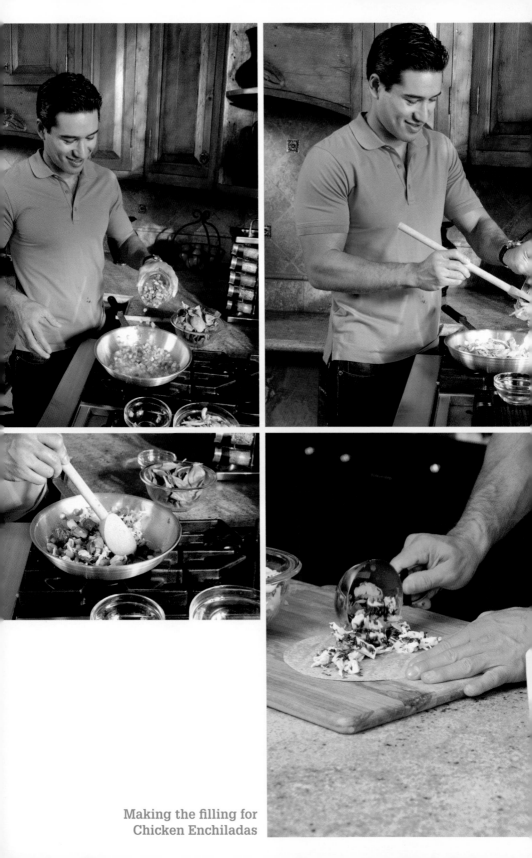

Making the filling for
Chicken Enchiladas

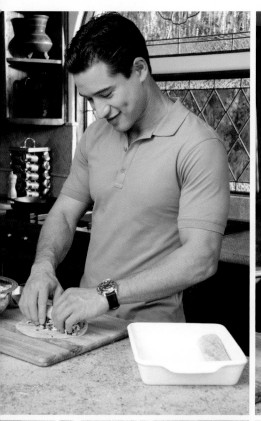
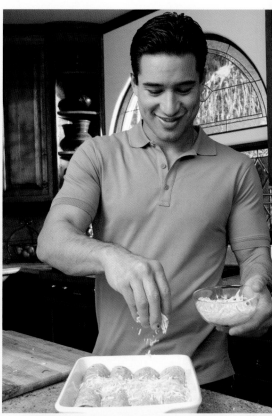
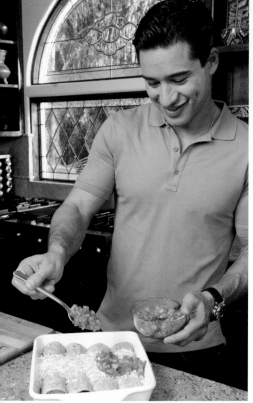
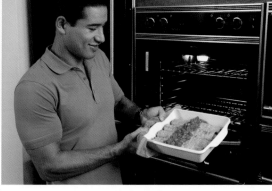

Rolling the enchiladas and
setting them up for the oven

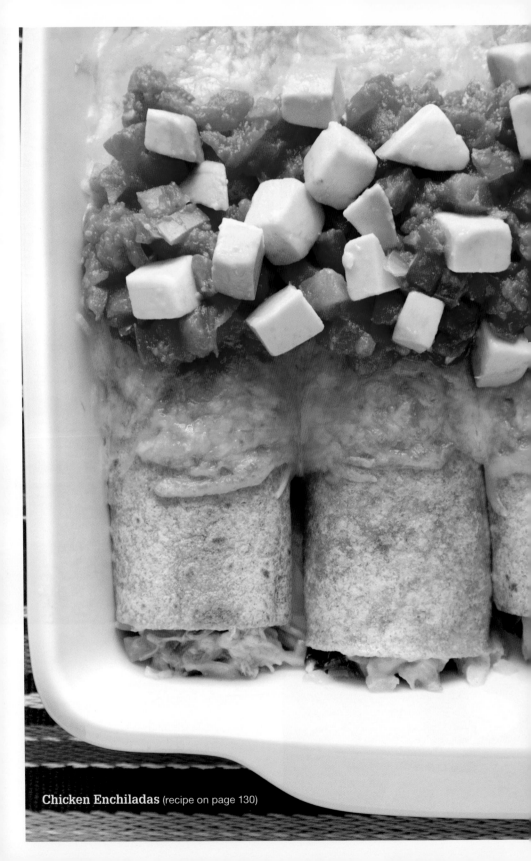

Chicken Enchiladas (recipe on page 130)

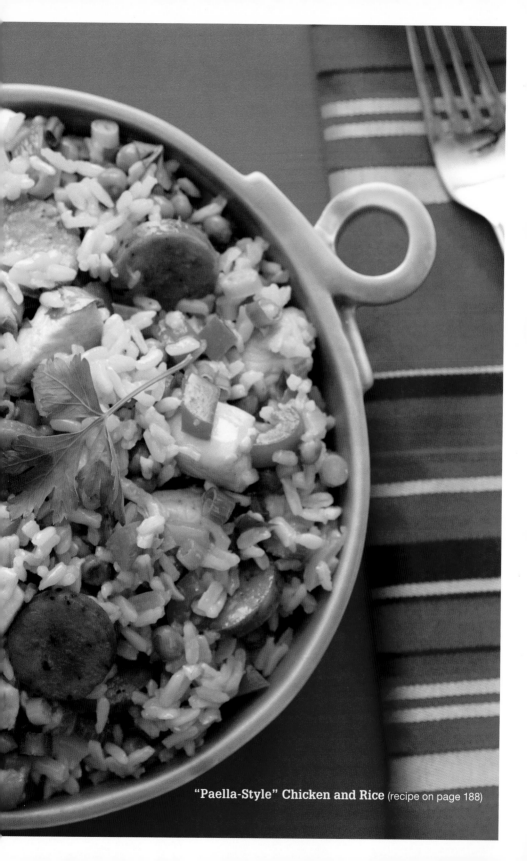

"Paella-Style" Chicken and Rice (recipe on page 188)

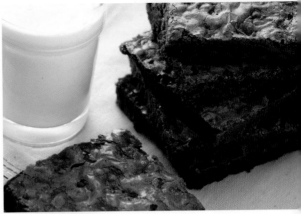

Dark Chocolate Brownies
(recipe on page 92)

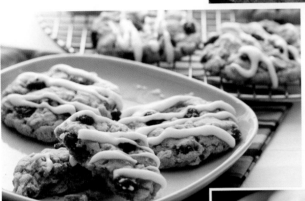

Oatmeal Raisin Cookies
(recipe on page 180)

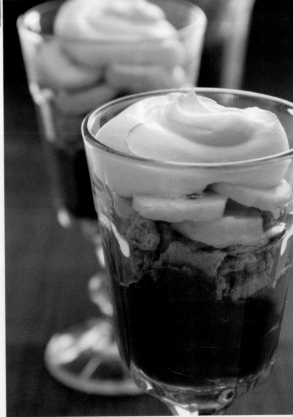

Ice Box Cake Parfaits
(recipe on page 171)

GROCERY LIST

▶ Produce

☐ Bananas: 14

☐ Apples: 12

☐ Melon: 1

☐ Blueberries: 2 pints

☐ Strawberries (fresh): 1 quart

☐ Oranges: 4

☐ Grapes: 1½ pounds

☐ Raisins: 1 small container

☐ Celery: 1 bunch

☐ Parsley: 1 bunch

☐ Cilantro: 1 bunch

☐ Lettuce (mixed greens or a combination of romaine and green leaf lettuces): 3 heads

☐ Baby carrots: 1 pound bag

☐ Cucumbers: 4 large

☐ Tomatoes: 5

☐ Onions: 2

☐ Garlic: 1 head

☐ Sweet potatoes: 4 small

☐ Broccoli: 1 bunch

☐ Scallions: 1 bunch

☐ Bell peppers: 3
(1 red and 2 any color)

☐ Asparagus: 2 bunches

☐ Lemons: 1

☐ Limes: 2

☐ Avocados: 3

☐ Orange juice: 2 half-gallon containers

▶ Dairy & Eggs

☐ Eggs: 1½ dozen

☐ Skim milk: 1 gallon

☐ Nonfat Greek yogurt:
6 large tubs

☐ Nonfat fruit yogurt:
4 6-ounce containers

☐ Unsalted butter: 1 stick

☐ Grated Parmesan cheese

☐ Shredded cheddar cheese:
1 package

☐ Finely shredded Mexican blend cheese: 1 package

☐ Low fat cheese: 16 slices

▶ Bakery

☐ Multigrain bread: 1 loaf

☐ Whole wheat pita: 4 each

☐ Whole wheat bread: 2 loaves

☐ Whole wheat English muffins: 4

☐ Whole wheat flour tortilla: 6

▶ Meat & Deli and Seafood

☐ Chicken breast (boneless, skinless): 3 pounds

- ☐ Rotisserie chicken: 1
- ☐ Low sodium turkey breast: 1 pound
- ☐ Pork tenderloin: 1 pound
- ☐ Andouille-flavored chicken sausage: 2 ounces
- ☐ Fresh cod: 1¼ pounds
- ☐ Shrimp, peeled and deveined (fresh or frozen): 1 pound
- ☐ Hummus: 2 large containers
- ☐ Cheese tortellini: 1 pound

▶ **Frozen**

- ☐ Frozen vegetables (like peas and carrots): 1 small package
- ☐ Frozen peas: 1 small package

▶ **Grocery & Pantry Items**

- ☐ Whole grain cereal: 1 box
- ☐ Cornflakes cereal: 1 box
- ☐ Rolled oats: 1 small canister
- ☐ Slivered almonds
- ☐ Salted cashews
- ☐ Whole wheat couscous
- ☐ Brown rice
- ☐ Barbecue sauce
- ☐ Rice vinegar
- ☐ Honey
- ☐ Mayonnaise
- ☐ Maple syrup
- ☐ Fruit spread
- ☐ Natural peanut butter
- ☐ Balsamic vinaigrette
- ☐ Low fat Ranch dressing

- ☐ Salsa
- ☐ Low sodium chicken broth
- ☐ Canned black beans: 1 15-ounce can
- ☐ Olive oil
- ☐ Canola oil
- ☐ Vanilla extract
- ☐ Saffron
- ☐ Curry powder
- ☐ Ground cumin
- ☐ Ground cinnamon
- ☐ Nonstick cooking spray
- ☐ Kosher salt
- ☐ Black pepper

Prep Day on Sunday:
- ▶ Make Chicken Salad
- ▶ Prepare chicken for meals on Thursday (or purchase a rotisserie chicken)
- ▶ Cook brown rice for Rice & Beans (Thursday night dinner)

Friday night's "make your own takeout" is fish sticks—a highly processed food option (usually comes boxed/frozen or deep fried at a restaurant). Forget the salty boxed fish sticks and make your own healthier and tastier version.

Whole grain cereal recommendations: Bran Flakes, Kashi Go Lean, or Nature's Path Multigrain Flakes

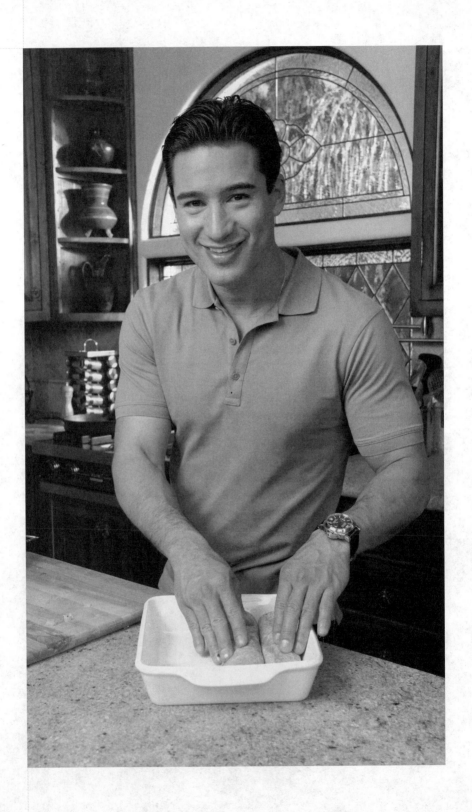

SUNDAY: "PREP DAY"

▶ **Cinnamon-Banana French Toast (see recipe on page 69)**
▶ **6 fl oz orange juice**

Calories: 452	**NUTRIENT INTAKE:**
Total Fat: 8.5g	Carbs 69%
Saturated Fat: 3g	Protein 14%
Carbohydrate: 80g	Fat 17%
Protein: 16g	
Sodium: 355mg	
Cholesterol: 117mg	
Fiber: 10g	

LUNCH

▶ **Turkey & Cheese Lettuce Cups:** 4 oz deli turkey breast, 2 slices low fat cheese, 1 tablespoon honey mustard, wrapped in Bibb or Romaine lettuce leaves

Double Duty Option:

▪ switch up your options—try roast beef with Swiss cheese and Ranch dressing

▶ **1 cup diced melon**

Calories: 438	**NUTRIENT INTAKE:**
Total Fat: 16g	Carbs 24%
Saturated Fat: 9.5g	Protein 40%
Carbohydrate: 25g	Fat 36%
Protein: 41g	
Sodium: 834mg	
Cholesterol: 85mg	
Fiber: 2.5g	

SNACK

▶ **1 cup grapes**

Calories: 110	**NUTRIENT INTAKE:**
Total Fat: 0g	Carbs 94%
Saturated Fat: 0g	Protein 4%
Carbohydrate: 29g	Fat 2%
Protein: 1g	
Sodium: 3mg	
Cholesterol: 0g	
Fiber: 1.5g	

"Paella-Style" Chicken and Rice

SERVES: 4

This simple rice dish has all the flavors of classic paella. If you can't find Andouille chicken sausage, use 1 ounce of Andouille pork sausage because it is higher in fat. If you don't like the taste of saffron, replace it with Italian seasoning for a completely different spin on this dish.

1 tablespoon olive oil
2 oz Andouille-flavored chicken sausage
½ cup chopped onion
½ cup chopped celery
½ teaspoon kosher salt
1 teaspoon saffron
1 cup brown rice (dry)
2 cups homemade (or store-bought, low sodium) chicken broth
1 pound boneless, skinless chicken breast, cut into large chunks
1 cup frozen peas, thawed
1 red bell pepper, thinly sliced
Chopped fresh parsley and scallions to taste

1. Heat oil in a large stockpot. Add chicken sausage and sauté for 2–3 minutes. Add onion and celery; season with salt and saffron. Add brown rice and chicken broth—stir well. Bring to a boil and add chunks of chicken. Cover and cook for 25–30 minutes or until all the liquid has been absorbed and the rice is tender. Stir in peas and sliced bell pepper. Serve in bowls, topped with parsley and scallions.

Calories: 425
Total Fat: 9g
Saturated Fat: 1.5g
Carbohydrate: 48g
Protein: 38g
Sodium: 518mg
Cholesterol: 81mg
Fiber: 4.5g

NUTRIENT INTAKE:

Carbs 45%
Protein 35%
Fat 20%

Extra Prep:

- Prepare the Chicken Salad with Fresh Herbs (page 133) for this week
- Prepare chicken for meals on Thursday (or purchase a rotisserie chicken)
- Cook brown rice for Rice & Beans (Thursday night dinner)

NUTRITION FOR THE DAY

Calories: 1427
Total Fat: 35g
Saturated Fat: 16g
Carbohydrate: 183g
Protein: 97g
Sodium: 1821mg
Cholesterol: 283mg
Fiber: 19g

NUTRIENT INTAKE:

Carbs 51%

Protein 27%

Fat 22%

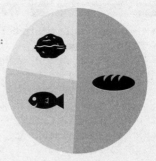

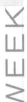
BREAKFAST

- ► 1½ cups whole grain cereal
- ► 1 cup skim milk
- ► ½ cup sliced strawberries

Calories: 311
Total Fat: 2g
Saturated Fat: 0.5g
Carbohydrate: 67g
Protein: 15g
Sodium: 400mg
Cholesterol: 5mg
Fiber: 12g

NUTRIENT INTAKE:

Carbs 78%
Protein 17%
Fat 5%

LUNCH

- ► 1 banana

► Chicken Tortellini Soup

SERVES: 4

6 cups homemade (or store-bought, low sodium) chicken broth
2 cups cooked cheese tortellini
2 cups frozen mixed vegetables (such as peas and carrots), thawed
¼ cup grated Parmesan cheese, divided
Chopped fresh parsley and ground black pepper to taste

1. Heat chicken broth in a large saucepan. Add tortellini and vegetables and simmer until heated through (about 5 minutes). Serve topped with 1 tablespoon grated cheese, parsley, and black pepper.

Double Duty Option:

- combine store-bought cheese tortellini with white beans, vegetables, chunks of cooked lean protein (chicken, shrimp, or pork tenderloin), a drizzle of olive oil, and fresh basil for a satisfying one-dish meal

Calories: 430
Total Fat: 9 g
Saturated Fat: 3.5g
Carbohydrate: 69g
Protein: 20g
Sodium: 679mg
Cholesterol: 30mg
Fiber: 7.5g

NUTRIENT INTAKE:

Carbs 63%
Protein 19%
Fat 18%

SNACK

▸ 8 oz nonfat Greek yogurt
▸ 1 tablespoon natural peanut butter

Double Duty Option:

- granola and a piece of fruit for on-the-go

Calories: 225
Total Fat: 8.5g
Saturated Fat: 1.5g
Carbohydrate: 12g
Protein: 23.5g
Sodium: 100mg
Cholesterol: 0mg
Fiber: 1.5g

NUTRIENT INTAKE:

Carbs 22%
Protein 43%
Fat 35%

DINNER

▸ Veggie Quesadillas (see recipe on page 104)

Double Duty Option:

- serve veggies and cheese rolled in the tortilla with some cooked brown rice for a veggie burrito
- 1 cup sliced cucumber topped with 1 tablespoon balsamic vinaigrette

Calories: 464
Total Fat: 26g
Saturated Fat: 8g
Carbohydrate: 38g
Protein: 20g
Sodium: 860mg
Cholesterol: 38mg
Fiber: 4g

NUTRIENT INTAKE:

Carbs 33%
Protein 17%
Fat 50%

NUTRITION FOR THE DAY

Calories: 1429
Total Fat: 45g
Saturated Fat: 14g
Carbohydrate: 188g
Protein: 79g
Sodium: 2297mg
Cholesterol: 73mg
Fiber: 26g

NUTRIENT INTAKE:

Carbs 51%
Protein 21%
Fat 28%

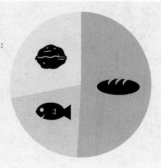

WEEK

BREAKFAST

- ▸ 2 tablespoons natural peanut butter
- ▸ 1 slice whole wheat bread
- ▸ 1 apple

Double Duty Option:

- swap out bread for a whole grain waffle

Calories: 363
Total Fat: 18g
Saturated Fat: 3g
Carbohydrate: 39g
Protein: 11g
Sodium: 166mg
Cholesterol: 0mg
Fiber: 12g

NUTRIENT INTAKE:

Carbs 43%

Protein 12%

Fat 45%

LUNCH

- ▸ Chicken Salad with Fresh Herbs (see recipe on page 133)
- ▸ 2 slices whole wheat bread

Double Duty Option:

- serve over mixed greens or in a whole wheat wrap

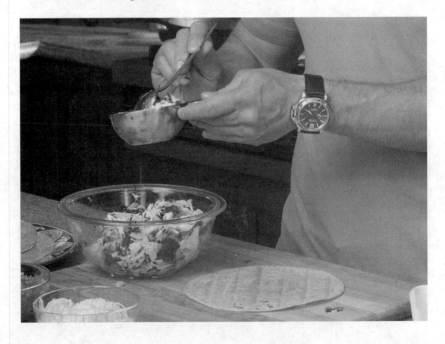

▶ **6 oz nonfat fruit yogurt**

Calories: 492
Total Fat: 10g
Saturated Fat: 1.5g
Carbohydrate: 58g
Protein: 42g
Sodium: 574mg
Cholesterol: 75mg
Fiber: 10g

NUTRIENT INTAKE:

Carbs 47%

Protein 35%

Fat 18%

SNACKS

▶ **10 baby carrots**
▶ **½ cup hummus**

Calories: 175
Total Fat: 6g
Saturated Fat: 0g
Carbohydrate: 24g
Protein: 5g
Sodium: 538mg
Cholesterol: 0mg
Fiber: 6g

NUTRIENT INTAKE:

Carbs 57%

Protein 11%

Fat 32%

DINNER

▶ **Curry-Roasted Shrimp with Cashew Couscous**
SERVES: 4

1 pound large shrimp (raw), peeled and deveined
2 teaspoons canola oil
1 teaspoon curry powder
¼ teaspoon kosher salt

1¼ cups homemade (or store-bought, low sodium) chicken broth
1 cup whole wheat couscous

> Whole wheat couscous is a delicious and super-quick
> cooking whole grain option.

¼ cup thinly sliced onion
½ cup raisins
¾ cup salted cashews
Chopped scallions and diced cucumber to taste

1. Preheat oven to 400 degrees F. Place shrimp on a baking sheet; toss with canola oil, curry powder, and salt. Roast for 3–4 minutes per side until cooked through. While the shrimp is cooking, bring the chicken broth to a boil in a medium saucepan. Stir in the couscous, onion, and raisins. Turn off heat, cover, and allow to sit for 10 minutes. Fluff with a fork and gently mix in cashews. Serve with roasted shrimp topped with chopped scallions and cucumber, if desired.

Calories: 512
Total Fat: 15.5g
Saturated Fat: 3g
Carbohydrate: 63g
Protein: 36g
Sodium: 582mg
Cholesterol: 175mg
Fiber: 5.5g

NUTRIENT INTAKE:

Carbs 47%

Protein 27%

Fat 26%

NUTRITION FOR THE DAY

Calories: 1540
Total Fat: 50g
Saturated Fat: 8g
Carbohydrate: 184g
Protein: 94g
Sodium: 1861mg
Cholesterol: 249mg
Fiber: 32g

NUTRIENT INTAKE:

Carbs 47%

Protein 24%

Fat 29%

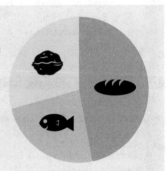

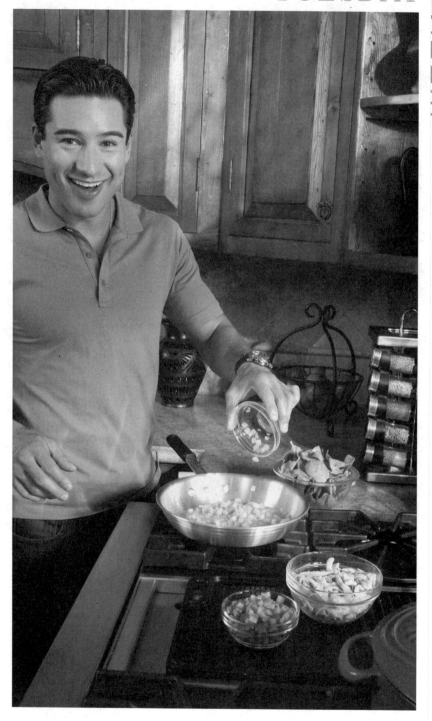

WEDNESDAY

BREAKFAST

- ▸ **1 cup nonfat Greek yogurt topped with**
- ▸ **¾ cup blueberries and 3 tablespoons slivered almonds**

Calories: 286
Total Fat: 11g
Saturated Fat: 1g
Carbohydrate: 24g
Protein: 25g
Sodium: 86mg
Cholesterol: 0mg
Fiber: 6g

NUTRIENT INTAKE:

Carbs 36%

Protein 33%

Fat 31%

LUNCH

- ▸ **Grilled Cheese & Tomato:** 2 slices of whole wheat bread, 2 slices low fat cheese, 2 slices of tomato, grilled in a nonstick pan

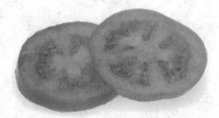

Double Duty Option:

- ▪ experiment with different types of cheese, add baby spinach, or thinly sliced bell pepper

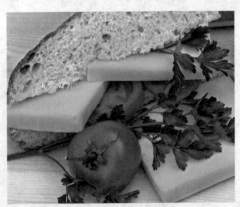

- ▸ **1 orange**

Calories: 327
Total Fat: 6g
Saturated Fat: 2.5g
Carbohydrate: 46g
Protein: 23g
Sodium: 619mg
Cholesterol: 12mg
Fiber: 11.5g

NUTRIENT INTAKE:

Carbs 55%
Protein 28%
Fat 17%

SNACK

▶ 8 oz nonfat Greek yogurt
▶ 1 tablespoon natural peanut butter

Double Duty Option:

▪ granola bar and a piece of fruit for on-the-go

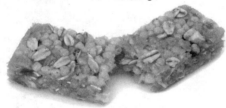

Calories: 225
Total Fat: 8.5g
Saturated Fat: 1.5g
Carbohydrate: 12g
Protein: 23.5g
Sodium: 100mg
Cholesterol: 0mg
Fiber: 1.5g

NUTRIENT INTAKE:

Carbs 22%
Protein 43%
Fat 35%

DINNER

▶ 4 oz roasted or grilled pork tenderloin

> Pork tenderloin is a tasty lean protein option—one of the best sources of the B vitamin, thiamin.

▶ 1 cup cooked asparagus
▶ 1 small baked sweet potato

> Sweet potato is less starchy than white potatoes and chock-full of the antioxidant beta-carotene.

Calories: 483
Total Fat: 9g
Saturated Fat: 3g
Carbohydrate: 60g
Protein: 46g
Sodium: 266mg
Cholesterol: 107mg
Fiber: 16g

NUTRIENT INTAKE:

Carbs 48%

Protein 36%

Fat 16%

DESSERT:

▶ **Kids Choice:** Any dessert recipe on the Extra Lean Family meal plan

NUTRITION FOR THE DAY

Calories: 1447
Total Fat: 38g
Saturated Fat: 8g
Carbohydrate: 165g
Protein: 119g
Sodium: 1128mg
Cholesterol: 129mg
Fiber: 35g

NUTRIENT INTAKE:

Carbs 45%

Protein 32%

Fat 23%

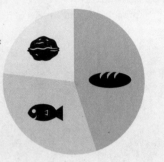

BREAKFAST

▸ 1 cup cooked oatmeal topped with 2 tablespoons raisins and a sprinkle of cinnamon
▸ 6 fl oz orange juice

Calories: 438
Total Fat: 3g
Saturated Fat: 0.5g
Carbohydrate: 73g
Protein: 8g
Sodium: 366mg
Cholesterol: 0mg
Fiber: 7g

NUTRIENT INTAKE:

Carbs 82%
Protein 9%
Fat 9%

LUNCH

Double Duty Option for Grilled Chicken Salsa and Veggies
▸ **Chicken Salsa Wraps:** Shredded cooked chicken with cheese, salsa, and lettuce in a whole wheat tortilla

> Salsa is a low calorie condiment and kicks up the flavor of chicken, rice, or egg dishes

OR

▸ **Grilled Chicken Salad:** 3 cups mixed greens topped with 4 oz grilled chicken, ⅓ cup diced avocado, 1 tablespoon salsa, 2 tablespoons shredded cheese, chopped tomato, and 2 teaspoons olive oil & lime juice to taste

> LEFTOVER TIP: Ripe tomato and creamy avocado on whole grain bread make a hunger-fighting sandwich.

Calories: 470
Total Fat: 28g
Saturated Fat: 7.5g
Carbohydrate: 14g
Protein: 42g
Sodium: 306mg
Cholesterol: 107mg
Fiber: 7.5g

NUTRIENT INTAKE:

Carbs 11%
Protein 37%
Fat 52%

SNACK

- ▶ 1 apple
- ▶ 1 tablespoon peanut butter or almond butter

Calories: 177
Total Fat: 9g
Saturated Fat: 1.5g
Carbohydrate: 22g
Protein: 4g
Sodium: 16mg
Cholesterol: 0mg
Fiber: 5g

NUTRIENT INTAKE:

Carbs 49%
Protein 8%
Fat 43%

DINNER

- ▶ BBQ Chicken with Rice & Beans (see recipe on page 70)
- ▶ Cucumber Salad (see recipe on page 71)

Calories: 521
Total Fat: 11g
Saturated Fat: 2g
Carbohydrate: 51g
Protein: 52g
Sodium: 320mg
Cholesterol: 120mg
Fiber: 6.5g

NUTRIENT INTAKE:

Carbs 40%
Protein 41%
Fat 19%

NUTRITION FOR THE DAY

Calories: 1503
Total Fat: 50g
Saturated Fat: 11.5g
Carbohydrate: 159g
Protein: 108g
Sodium: 791mg
Cholesterol: 239mg
Fiber: 25g

NUTRIENT INTAKE:

Carbs 45%
Protein 28%
Fat 27%

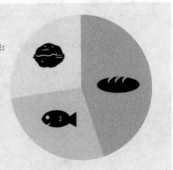

BREAKFAST

▶ **Rise & Shine Smoothie** (see recipe on page 86)

Double Duty Option:

▪ swap orange juice with mango or pineapple juice for a tropical flavor.

Calories: 274
Total Fat: 0g
Saturated Fat: 0g
Carbohydrate: 58g
Protein: 13g
Sodium: 44mg
Cholesterol: 0mg
Fiber: 4g

NUTRIENT INTAKE:

Carbs 80%
Protein 18%
Fat 2%

LUNCH

▶ **Peanut Butter & Jam:** 2 slices whole wheat bread topped with 2 tablespoons peanut butter and 1 tablespoon fruit spread
▶ **8 fl oz skim milk**

Double Duty Option:

▪ experiment with cashew or sunflower butter instead of peanut butter.

Calories: 497
Total Fat: 19.5g
Saturated Fat: 3g
Carbohydrate: 56g
Protein: 23g
Sodium: 431mg
Cholesterol: 5mg
Fiber: 11g

NUTRIENT INTAKE:

Carbs 46%
Protein 19%
Fat 35%

SNACK

▶ **10 baby carrots**
▶ **½ cup hummus**

Calories: 175
Total Fat: 6g
Saturated Fat: 0g
Carbohydrate: 24g
Protein: 5g
Sodium: 538mg
Cholesterol: 0mg
Fiber: 6g

NUTRIENT INTAKE:

Carbs 57%
Protein 11%
Fat 32%

DINNER

▶ **Homemade Fish Sticks**

SERVES: 4

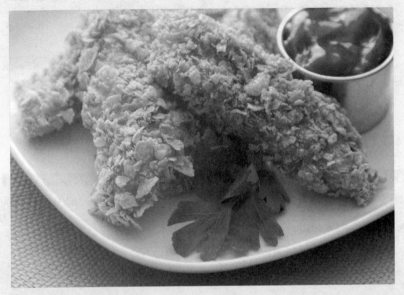

3 egg whites
3 cups cornflakes cereal
¼ teaspoon kosher salt
¼ teaspoon black pepper
1¼ pounds fresh cod, cut into strips

Cod is a mild and tender, low-mercury fish—perfect for fish sticks.

1. Preheat oven to 400 degrees F. Spray a baking sheet with nonstick spray and set aside. Place egg whites in a bowl and beat well. Place cereal in plastic bag; season with salt and pepper and crush well. Dredge fish in egg whites and place in bag to coat with cereal; transfer to baking sheet. Bake for 8 to 10 minutes per side, or until fish is cooked through.

Double Duty Option:
  ▪ leave fish filets whole and serve with a mixture of Greek yogurt and chili sauce for a spicy topping

OR

  ▪ make parchment paper sacks filled with fresh herbs, sliced onion, and pieces of cod and bake at 400 degrees F for 20–30 minutes

▶ 1 cup steamed broccoli topped with 1 teaspoon olive oil and lemon juice
▶ 2 cups mixed greens with 1 tablespoon Ranch dressing

Calories: 502
Total Fat: 14g
Saturated Fat: 2g
Carbohydrate: 54g
Protein: 40g
Sodium: 460mg
Cholesterol: 77mg
Fiber: 7g

NUTRIENT INTAKE:

Carbs 43%

Protein 33%

Fat 25%

NUTRITION FOR THE DAY

Calories: 1445
Total Fat: 40g
Saturated Fat: 5.5g
Carbohydrate: 192g
Protein: 81g
Sodium: 1448mg
Cholesterol: 81mg
Fiber: 28g

NUTRIENT INTAKE:

Carbs 43%

Protein 22%

Fat 25%

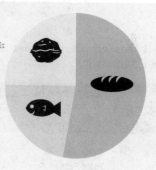

BREAKFAST

▸ **2 eggs, scrambled with ½ cup vegetables**

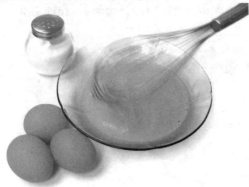

▸ **1 toasted whole wheat English muffin**
▸ **1 banana**

Banana provides your daily dose of potassium for healthy muscles.

Calories: 395
Total Fat: 11.5g
Saturated Fat: 3.5g
Carbohydrate: 56g
Protein: 20g
Sodium: 374mg
Cholesterol: 323mg
Fiber: 7g

NUTRIENT INTAKE:

Carbs 55%

Protein 20%

Fat 25%

LUNCH

▸ **Avocado & Tomato Salad:** 3 cups mixed greens topped with 2 oz grilled chicken or turkey breast, ½ avocado (sliced), ½ cup diced tomato

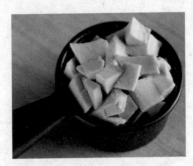

► 2 tablespoons low fat Ranch dressing
► 1 cup strawberries

Calories: 538
Total Fat: 21.5g
Saturated Fat: 8g
Carbohydrate: 25g
Protein: 5g
Sodium: 602mg
Cholesterol: 124mg
Fiber: 8g

NUTRIENT INTAKE:

Carbs 32%
Protein 7%
Fat 61%

SNACK

► 1 apple

Calories: 72
Total Fat: 0g
Saturated Fat: 0g
Carbohydrate: 19g
Protein: 0g
Sodium: 1mg
Cholesterol: 0g
Fiber: 3g

NUTRIENT INTAKE:

Carbs 95%
Protein 3%
Fat 2%

DINNER

► **Flatbreads:** 1 whole wheat pita topped with 3 oz cooked chicken breast (from a rotisserie chicken or leftover BBQ chicken), ¼ cup shredded cheddar cheese and sliced peppers; bake until cheese is melted

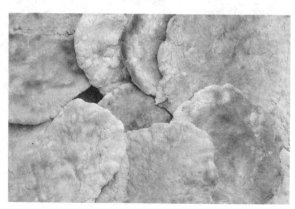

Double Duty Option:

▪ mix up the toppings with broccoli or asparagus

Calories: 435
Total Fat: 14g
Saturated Fat: 6g
Carbohydrate: 40g
Protein: 34g
Sodium: 596mg
Cholesterol: 102mg
Fiber: 6g

NUTRIENT INTAKE:

Carbs 36%

Protein 36%

Fat 28%

DESSERT

▶ **Special Treat:** Go out for ice cream for a scoop each or stop by the local bakery and get a family favorite—just keep the portions under control.

NUTRITION FOR THE DAY

Calories: 1544
Total Fat: 48g
Saturated Fat: 18g
Carbohydrate: 160g
Protein: 70g
Sodium: 1600mg
Cholesterol: 471mg
Fiber: 24g

NUTRIENT INTAKE:

Carbs 47%

Protein 21%

Fat 32%

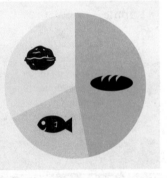

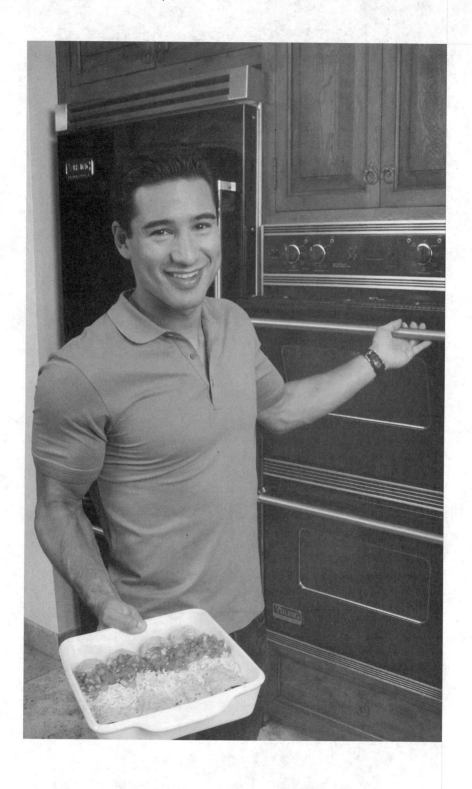

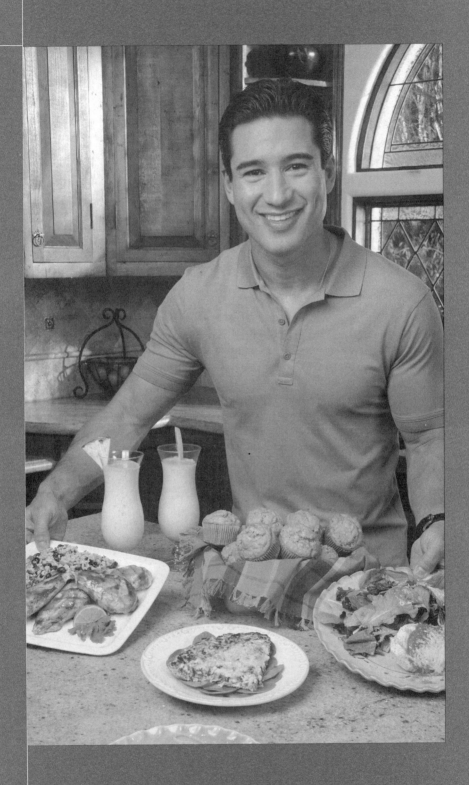

5.

extra lean family
nutrition for happy and healthy kids

Don't you wish that every child came with his own little instruction manual? While I may not be able to help you answer those tough parenting questions such as why your contented daughter is now a surly teen who rolls her eyes every time you look at her, I can tell you that there is some good, solid, essential information available to understand your children's health and nutrition. In this chapter, I've rounded up what I think is the most important *Extra Lean Family* nutrition information so that you can understand just what kind of food—and how much—your growing child needs to be healthy and happy.

What Every Parent Should Know about Children and Food

1. GROWING BODIES NEED MORE CALORIES AND CARBOHYDRATES FOR ENERGY

With childhood obesity in the media spotlight, restricting calories for kids would seem like the logical fix. However, that couldn't be further from a long-term solution. If there's one underlying and overwhelming theme that I want you to take away from this book, it's that kids have no business being on "diets." They need to be kids. They need to be moving their bodies, burning energy, and eating healthy carbs to fuel their activities every day of the week.

BOYS TYPICALLY GROW 9 inches during their teen years, while girls often begin a rapid growth spurt between the ages of ten and fourteen, adding on 7 inches in those three years. During this time, their calorie needs soar—and so does their need for a wide variety of nutrients.

No wonder I ate all of those tortillas with butter when I came home from school! Like many kids, I didn't really care—or notice—whether the food I was eating was high in calories or had any nutritional value beyond filling my belly.

The best kinds of healthy carbs are grains, fruits, and veggies. Half of your children's grain servings should be whole wheat, oats, or another unrefined type, because unrefined grains convey bigger amounts of important nutrients like vitamin E, fiber, and magnesium. These whole grains can also reduce the risk of your children suffering health risks from diabetes, asthma, or heart disease later in life. Switch picky eaters gradually by using breads that are a mix of whole and refined grains.

How many servings:

Toddlers 3
Preschoolers 4–5
Older kids and teens 4–5

EXTRA LEAN FACT

A RESEARCH STUDY of children ages eight to thirteen found that children who ate whole grains were 54 percent less likely to have asthma—possibly because whole grains are packed with antioxidants that may keep airways from becoming inflamed.

Kids need fruits and vegetables for their unique disease-fighting compounds, maybe even more than adults do. Try to divide your children's servings between the two, aiming to have them eat at least a single serving of particularly powerful orange or dark green vegetables every day, like carrots or broccoli.

How many servings:

Toddlers 4
Preschoolers 4–6
Older kids and teens 5–7

2. CALCIUM DOES A BODY GOOD

Children need 500mg of calcium between the ages of one and three; older children need 800mg daily to ensure that they build strong bones and teeth. If your child is a milk lover, it's easy; otherwise, choose low fat yogurt, fortified fruit juice, or cheese. Many breads contain vitamin D.

How many servings:

Toddlers 2–3
Preschoolers 3–4
Older children and teens 4

 EXTRA LEAN FACT A RECENT STUDY revealed that people who consumed the most calcium as children lowered their chances of suffering a stroke as adults.

3. FATS PROTECT CHILDREN'S HEALTH

Did you know that even children can get high cholesterol? Unsaturated fats, like peanuts and olive oil, can help keep cholesterol low for kids as well as adults. Fats are also important for children because they provide vitamin E and transport vitamins in the body. Remember that nuts are choking hazards for kids under age three. Simply by switching from butter to olive or canola oil when you cook can go a long way toward lessening the chance that your child will be obese or suffer from high cholesterol.

How many servings:

Toddlers 3
Preschoolers 3–4
Older kids and teens 4–5

4. CHILDREN NEED EXTRA PROTEIN DURING PERIODS OF RAPID GROWTH

By now you know I'm a big fan of protein. Protein is super healthy and is critical for growing kids. This is especially true during growth spurts and times when your child is very physically active. I know that whenever I had a tough wrestling match in high school, I'd come home sore and exhausted. I craved protein after working out, and now I know why. A child's growing body, specifically the muscle cells, requires an enormous amount of protein synthesis, and the more protein available to synthesize, the better his body can grow and mature. Plus, proteins pack an additional punch by providing nutrients like iron, zinc, and B vitamins. Shop for lean meats, like beef with "loin" or "round" in the name, and take the skin off poultry and turkey. Your children will also benefit from eating fish and beans at least once a week, because these foods have nutrients you can't get anywhere else.

How many servings:

Toddlers 2
Preschoolers 2–4
Older children and teens 3–5

WHAT IF MY CHILD WON'T EAT MEAT?

Lots of younger children go through phases where they won't touch meat. Some don't like the texture, while others would just rather chew something else. And many middle schoolers and high schoolers decide to become vegetarians all on their own, even if Mom and Dad are meat lovers. Children can certainly be healthy on a well-planned vegetarian diet. In fact, children who avoid meat are often taking in less harmful saturated fat while eating more fresh vegetables and fiber than their meat-eating pals. They tend to have lower cholesterol levels and are leaner, too. The important thing is to make sure that vegetarian kids get the same important mix of nutrients. Here's how you can replace what's missing if your child doesn't eat meat:

Iron	Serve foods rich in vitamin C (like strawberries, broccoli, and oranges) with beans, spinach, whole wheat bread (the vitamin C will boost iron absorption)
Protein	Soy-based veggie burgers or other foods, nuts, nut butters
Vitamin B12	Dairy products, fortified cereals
Zinc	Almonds, tofu, wheat germ added to muffins or smoothies

5. ALL KIDS NEED A BALANCE OF MACRONUTRIENTS

I've made a big deal about protein for growth spurts and working muscles, but you can't forget about the balance factor. I've stressed it before, spreading the love to all sorts of foods, but variety is absolutely necessary. Not simply to tempt the taste buds of everyone at the table, although that's one nice thing about having a diverse menu, but because eating the same foods day in and day out means that you're probably deficient in any number of important nutrients. By enlarging the radius, exposing yourself and family to many kinds of foods, you increase the probability that everyone will get the right mix of vitamins and nutrients essential for overall health.

6. NUTRIENT-DENSE FOODS ARE KEY

While there is certainly room in my meal plan for the occasional sweet treat, your child's intake of so-called "empty" calories from candy, soda, and other junk foods should be moderate to low. The great thing about the meals is that all of them are packed with nutrients. You want your child's body to benefit from everything he consumes. This means avoiding foods that add calories and not much more. Good foods going in means healthy skin, growing bones and muscles and, most of all, energy to fuel all the processes, both internal and external, that a growing child needs.

7. FOOD ALLERGIES CAN JEOPARDIZE YOUR CHILD'S HEALTH

My sister is one of my best friends, and we've always played a big role in each other's lives. Even now, she lives just five minutes away from me and our families spend a lot of time together. My sister is a great mom, and I've loved being an uncle to her three kids—it was great practice for having a child of my own!

From watching my sister raise her kids and talking to our own pediatrician now about Gia Francesca, I know that food allergies are a real worry for a lot of parents. In fact, about six percent of kids suffer from them, and kids with food allergies are constantly having to be careful not to come into contact with foods that can make them sick, or even kill them. The foods most likely to cause allergic reactions in children include cow's milk, fish, wheat, soy, shellfish, and—the biggest culprit of all—nuts.

So, despite the fact that a peanut butter and jelly sandwich sounds as American as apple pie, many school cafeterias have banned peanuts, tree nuts, and any packaged foods that may have come into contact with

nuts during production. While all food allergies can be serious, causing symptoms that range from an upset stomach to vomiting and diar-
rhea, nut allergies are usually the most severe, leading to illness or even
death from anaphylactic shock, which basically causes kids to suffocate
if they're not treated soon enough.

Because infants and toddlers have immature immune and digestive
systems, most doctors—including our own—suggest that you wait until
your baby is around six months old to introduce solid foods. That way,
you'll reduce the likelihood that your child will suffer from food allergies. They also advise not giving peanuts or tree nuts to kids under age
three, especially if there's a family history of allergies. That's because
most kids have less severe allergic reactions, or outgrow them entirely,
if they're older.

8. INTRODUCING VARIETY EARLY IS THE KEY TO GOOD EATING HABITS

Ideally, I would like to have three kids of my own someday, but I might
even be up for more. No matter how many children I have, though, it's
going to be so much fun teaching them about all of the good foods there
are in the world.

I plan to start introducing Gia Francesca to lots of different kinds of
foods as soon as her doctor says it's okay. That's because I know from
my own childhood experiences that a child's earliest months and years
of eating with her family have a lasting influence on how she eats for life.

Gia Francesca has already learned so much. Even at two months,
she's smiling and following us around the kitchen with her eyes, and I
swear she's trying to talk to us with those cute sounds she makes. She's
already a really social baby, and we encourage that by talking to her
and acting like we're answering her questions when she babbles. Even
though she can't actually say any words, I know that she's busy trying to
figure out what words mean, and I think she understands a lot of what
we say already.

If she can do all of this now, I can't wait to see what Gia Francesca
will know what to do by the time she's older and eating solid foods. I
think food will be a great way for her to learn about textures and tastes,

of course, but maybe also about how much joy there is in looking at bright colors. Her taste buds are developing and she'll be curious, like all kids, so she'll be more willing to eat different foods as a baby than she will be when she's one of those two-year-olds whose favorite word is "no!"

My plan is to feed Gia Francesca something bright in addition to something green at every meal. I bet she'll have lots of fun trying everything from tomatoes and watermelon to carrots, sweet potatoes, and berries. Try this with your baby, too. As long as you mash or cut the food up into tiny pieces, you can feed your baby almost everything your family is eating on the meal plan.

MAKE YOUR OWN BABY FOOD

We owe it to our babies to give them the best possible start in life. It's never too early to introduce healthy eating habits in your child. Instead of spending money on prepackaged baby foods, you should try to make your own.

I use some jarred organic baby food for Gia Francesca when I'm looking for convenience. But I also love making her food myself. With the help of my trusty blender, I teach Gia Francesca to love the same healthy produce, grains, and meat that her mom and I enjoy. I'm hoping that Gia Francesca will already develop a love for good food before she's even out of diapers. Meanwhile, I'll know exactly what nutrients are fueling her, and I can have the pleasure of introducing my daughter to a huge variety of nutritious foods that aren't typically found in the baby food aisle of my grocery store.

As Gia Francesca's pediatrician advised, you should wait until your baby is around six months old before introducing solid foods. Your doctor will probably tell you the same thing, and will probably also want you to wait a few days after introducing each new kind of food to make sure that your baby doesn't have an allergic reaction to anything she eats. Most parents start babies on rice cereal, followed by oatmeal, mashed yellow vegetables, mashed green vegetables, and then pureed fruit.

As babies get a little older, they can start eating foods with bigger chunks. I was always amazed by my sister's kids, who ate practically everything even before they had teeth! Those gums were really hard!

It might seem intimidating to make food for your baby, but really, all you need at home is a blender or a food processor. To fix vegetables for your baby is easy, because you just do it the same way you would for yourself, steaming them on the stove or cooking them in the microwave. Just cook them longer so that they're soft enough to puree. Once the vegetables are soft, pour off some of the cooking water before you puree it, or the veggies will be watery. For young babies, the food should be the consistency of applesauce.

If you're giving fruit to your baby, not all of it has to be cooked first— you need to cook it only to soften it. Bananas can go into the blender right after you peel them. Wash blueberries, peaches, plums, and melons, and then you can slice and puree them without having to cook them first. Don't serve strawberries to your baby until she's at least a year old—a lot of babies are allergic to them. And, for fruits that are harder, like apples and pears, you should peel them and cook them before you stick those in the blender. Don't ever add sugar to the fruits; they have natural sweeteners, and your baby will already love them.

You can grind millet and quinoa in your food mill after you cook them. For meat, remove the skin and trim the fat, then cook it and blend it with a little liquid. Once your baby has had a good variety of foods and is a little older, you can also start blending pretty much anything your family is eating—soups, stews, casseroles—to feed your baby. It's a myth that babies don't like adventurous flavors!

After you've prepared your baby's food, pour it into an ice cube tray and freeze it. Then you can pop out the little cubes of food and store them in a freezer bag—just make sure to label the bags so that you know what's in them! Fruits and vegetables frozen this way can last six months. Frozen cubes of meat, poultry, and fish can last a month.

Super Healthy Foods for Kids

The minute I knew I was going to be a father, I made sure to be on top of what foods to provide my child so she can grow up healthy and happy. Now that you know the most important basic nutrition for kids, here's a list of "Super Healthy Foods." I call them that because kids love them, and because they provide super nutritional value. Once you and your kids discover how good they taste, and how much better you all feel after eating these particular foods, you'll start craving them instead of those sweet and salty goodies that pack on the pounds without giving your body the real fuel it needs to go on. You can also find these foods in the five-week meal plan:

Salmon: Salmon is packed with those heart-healthy omega-3 fats, which I talk about in this chapter as being important to boost your child's brain development and immune system. If your child won't eat salmon straight up, try glazing salmon fillets with orange juice or serve salmon burgers.

Blueberries: What kid doesn't love blueberry pancakes or blueberry muffins? And that's great news for parents, because blueberries are ranked among the healthiest foods you can eat. Blueberries are chock-full of antioxidants, and they help fight heart disease and diabetes. Some experts even say blueberries can protect against the toxic belly fat that's linked to obesity. Besides making blueberry pancakes, toss blueberries onto cereal and salads, or make blueberry ice pops by freezing blended blueberries and vanilla low fat yogurt.

Black Beans: You'll find black beans in a lot of the meals. That's because I can't say enough about what a great source of protein, fiber, and calcium they are—and kids need a lot of all three. Black beans also help guard your family against high cholesterol—something that kids can be at risk for, too. If your child won't eat black beans, try blending them and adding them to hummus or throw a few into quesadillas you make with low fat cheese.

Nonfat Greek Yogurt: I love Greek yogurt, not just for the taste, but because it has healthy bacteria that boost immunity and help digestion. Greek yogurt also has up to three times as much protein as and less sugar than regular yogurt. For kids, add a tiny bit of honey or maple syrup, and they'll crave it like it's a dessert.

Tomatoes: If your children love pasta with tomato sauce, that's great, because tomatoes are loaded with a cancer-fighting substance called lycopene. Even better news: cooking tomatoes makes them even healthier, because the heat helps release the lycopene. Add tomato sauce to turkey meatballs, or give your family pizza with tomato sauce and low fat cheese.

Tofu: Yeah, I know. I never ate tofu as a kid, either. But whole soy foods are such a great source of protein and cancer-fighting nutrients that it's worth trying to introduce tofu to your family if you don't already eat it. Dice and toss tofu into soups or stir-fries, and your kids may surprise you and gobble it down.

Cinnamon: This is a mighty spice and kids love it. Just a half teaspoon per day can lower LDL cholesterol, and studies show that cinnamon can aid in the prevention of diabetes. You can sprinkle cinnamon on your child's yogurt or cereal, or toss a teaspoon into pancakes and oatmeal. Some kids even love it on popcorn.

Cocoa: Chocolate? How can that be healthy? Luckily for parents, cocoa is definitely a Super Healthy Food for kids. That's because cocoa powder has one of the highest concentrations of a special compound that can lower blood pressure and boost heart health—a compound called "flavonoids." Flavonoids may also protect your child's skin from sun damage. Just make sure that you use at least 70 percent pure cocoa and that it isn't processed with alkali.

Besides serving cups of hot chocolate made the old-fashioned way, you can sprinkle cocoa on pancakes or French toast, or melt dark chocolate and dunk bananas and strawberries into it as a treat.

Great Snacks for Children

In Chapter One, you learned the importance of eating frequently to boost your metabolism, because your body will start shutting down if you hold back on the fuel you need, leaving you without the energy you need to work, study, or play. This is even truer for kids than it is for adults, because kids burn so many calories just by growing—plus, they're often in motion, even if they're just jiggling their knees under the table like I always used to do.

Making sure that your kids have healthy snacks is essential for keeping your kid's energy high, and can help you curb your child's unhealthy eating in between meals. Here are some of my top choices for kid snacks:

Baby carrots. Steam carrots until soft and cut into small pieces for babies and toddlers. Pack these beta-carotene-rich veggies in sealed plastic bags for older kids to take to school or to eat as snacks in the car.

Baked potatoes: Potatoes are loaded with potassium, rich in fiber, and lower in fat than regular greasy fries. If your child has a microwave at school, you can even bake them ahead of time and just have him heat them up when he's ready for a snack. Great when topped with nutritious chili, beans, broccoli, or low fat cheese.

Breakfast cereal: If your kids refuse to eat cereal that isn't sugary, combine sweet brands with less sugary varieties. Breakfast cereal is a surefire kiddie crowd pleaser and it's usually fortified with vitamins and minerals. It packs an extra nutritional punch with milk.

Broccoli: Calcium and vitamins infuse every bite of broccoli, and most kids will eat it if it's steamed bright green. If they won't touch the green stuff, get playful: make a broccoli face on pizza or plant a broccoli tree in a potato. You can also shave broccoli into soups.

Eggs: One scrambled egg will go a long way toward giving your child the essential protein and vitamin D he needs to build and repair muscles, and to help his body absorb calcium.

Orange juice: This is the most nutritious of all juices, plus O.J. is packed with potassium, vitamin C, and folate. If your child doesn't like milk, give him calcium-fortified orange juice.

Peanut butter: A good source of fiber, peanut butter is rich in protein, too. It makes a great dip for banana chunks, apple slices, and carrots. Use the less sugary natural peanut butter.

Pizza: Sure, it's one of their favorite junk foods, but pizza also can give your child healthy doses of grains, dairy, and vegetables. Choose pizza with low fat cheese and vegetables, and limit it to one slice.

Tortillas: Low fat wheat tortillas can be baked to make low fat chips, rolled up with turkey, or topped with low fat melted cheese for great quickie snacks.

Yogurt: Other than milk, yogurt probably gets more calcium into your child than any other food. Look for brands with live and active cultures; those have the bacteria necessary to keep intestines healthy. Be sure to look for brands with less sugar, or dilute sweet yogurts with plain yogurt. Also, try to stick to nonfat yogurt.

Cheese: Cheese is concentrated milk, really, made by mixing milk with enzymes to form solids. There are low fat versions of the cheeses most popular with kids, like American, mozzarella, cheddar, and Colby. And one ounce of low fat cheese—that's about four dice-sized cubes—can provide your child with the same amount of calcium, protein, and phosphorus as a cup of milk. Cheese can also help prevent cavities because it helps restore tooth enamel, and reduced-fat cheese can save your child from eating the saturated fats in many other protein sources they might otherwise go for, like hamburgers.

Children and Food Habits

So far, I've focused my attention in this chapter on providing you with the key information every parent should know about what foods children need, and how much, to provide the right number of calories and the best balance of protein, carbohydrates, and fats for children to be healthy and happy. However, a lot of parents may be tempted to ignore this information because they think it's too late for their family to undo bad eating habits. "If only I'd started giving my daughter healthy whole grain breads and fruit instead of cookies, she might be a healthy eater now instead of so overweight," one busy worried mom told me recently.

It's true that researchers have found that eating habits from childhood can definitely carry over into adulthood. For instance, if you reward your child with a sugary treat every time she hurts herself or reaches a goal, your child will come to view sugary treats as comfort foods. Imagine your sweet toddler as a college student. What will she do if she's depressed or bombs an exam? She'll reach for a cookie or a brownie, instead of exercising to improve her mood.

Luckily, it isn't ever too late for a child (or an adult!) to change his attitude toward food and adopt new and healthier ways to eat. Below, I've listed some tips to help you break down your child's bad food habits, whether he's six or sixteen.

How to Curb Constant Munching: While it's true that eating many small meals during the day is preferable to sitting down for three large ones, it's equally true that children who constantly munch and nibble won't learn to recognize feelings of hunger. All kids thrive on structure, so try to serve snacks and meals at about the same time every day. If he complains that he's hungry, remind him to wait ten minutes to see if he really is hungry. Chances are, he'll forget all about it. In addition, if you make sure to use the high-powered snacks included in our meal plan, your child will have enough protein and unsaturated fat to make him less likely to nibble between snacks and meals because he'll be more satisfied.

How to Prevent Sugar Overload: Babies have a natural love of sweet things. Unfortunately, the kind of sugar added to many desserts and sweet snacks will provide your child with lots of empty calories and very little nutrition. Establish some rules without depriving your child of treats. A good start is to limit sweets to once a day. Avoid fights by asking your child when he wants his treat—after school or after dinner?—so that he feels like he has a choice. Meanwhile, read food labels to see how much sugar is in foods that might seem healthy to you, like cereals, and avoid automatically offering dessert after every meal. Or, if your child insists on dessert, try healthier options, like bananas sprinkled with cinnamon or strawberries with fat-free whipped topping.

How to Add Veggies: Studies show that children who grow up eating vegetables will be more likely to eat vegetables as adults. Pressuring kids to eat vegetables leads to power struggles, however, so focus on making them tempting. Add a little reduced-fat shredded cheese, hummus, natural peanut butter, or low fat Ranch dressing for dipping to make vegetables more palatable to picky eaters. Children are also more likely to eat vegetables if you let them help arrange them on a tray, grow them in your garden, or cook them.

How to Curb Carbs: Certain kids seem to live on mac 'n' cheese or refuse to eat anything that isn't white. The problem is that, if they're gobbling down carbs in the form of white bread or noodles, their bodies will digest that food quickly and they'll be hungry again soon. Plus, they're not getting the nutrients they need from other foods. Many children don't like meat because it's too tough, but if you grill your meats or poach your poultry, your child will be more likely to eat it. You can also hide ground turkey in spaghetti sauce or dice chicken into soup. If your child still won't eat meat, upgrade

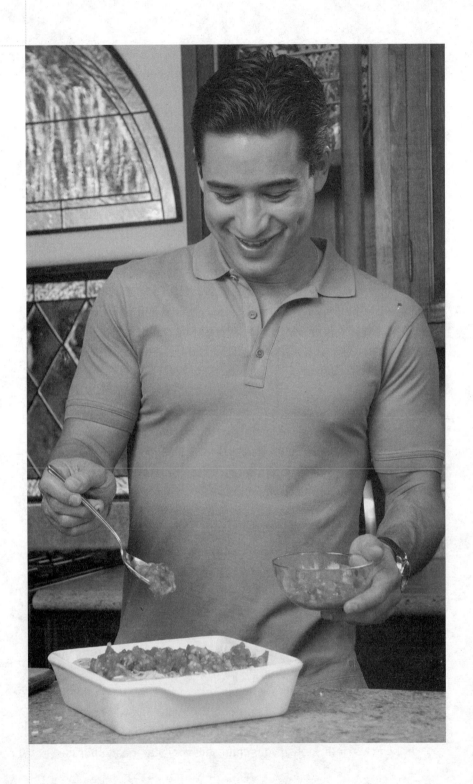

extra lean FAMILY

her carbs to whole grains and add other great protein sources like low fat dairy products, eggs, and beans.

How to Cut Back on Juice & Soda: Never, ever have soda in the house, and try to model good drinking habits; for instance, if your toddler sees you drinking water, she'll be more likely to want water with her meal. The same goes for soda! Always offer water first when your child is thirsty, and milk otherwise. While a small amount of natural, 100 percent juice is okay for kids, drinking more than half a cup will cause them to be too full to eat more nutritious foods. In addition, many juices are high in calories—there are 110 calories in a cup of apple juice—so that can add up quickly if your child is swilling juice all day long. You can get around this by diluting juice by at least half. For older kids and teens, adding seltzer can give them the pleasure of a fizzy drink without the high sugar content of soda.

How to Energize Young Athletes with the Right Foods: After my mom got me involved at the Boys & Girls Club, I never stopped moving. Wrestling, dancing, playing kickball or basketball: if there was a game, I was up for it. I loved to compete. And when I came home, I was starving. I ate anything and everything. I'd walk in the door and eat my grandmother's tortillas slathered in butter, down a couple of glasses of whole milk, then open the fridge and grab whatever was in there. I couldn't get enough food.

The thing is, I didn't really know back then what kind of foods would be the best to energize me as a young athlete. I didn't even think about nutrition. I just wanted to stop feeling hungry. I had no idea that I should be having protein at every meal in order to keep my energy level high and build up my muscles.

I want to help you teach your kids what I know now: that there are certain types of foods they should eat before and after a game or a practice that will really help them do their personal best. Whether your child is off to the State Championship cross-country meet or just kicking the soccer ball around the yard with friends, he needs the right foods to boost his performance. To give your young athletes the energy they need, try these strategies:

Serve a mini meal an hour before playtime. Be sure that it has lean protein and is easy to digest. Choices like a turkey and low fat cheese wrap sandwich or a small fruit-and-yogurt smoothie are always popular starters.

During sports practices and games, be sure that your child has snacks and water for breaks. Kids don't need sports drinks, unless they're really exerting themselves or it's an incredibly hot day, and they certainly shouldn't have any drink with caffeine. It's also a good idea for your child to have a halftime snack that will boost her energy and keep her hydrated. Ideal choices are granola bars and some orange slices.

After the game, give her a meal that's high in protein and carbs, plus water. Adding more protein and carbs to her daily intake after she's been expending energy on the field or basketball court will help your aspiring athlete to heal and rebuild her muscles. If it's a while before her next meal, give your athlete a simple snack. Even something as simple as chocolate milk has a nice balance of carbs, protein, and fluid. For her meal, try spaghetti and meat sauce with carrot sticks on the side, or a peanut butter and jelly sandwich with slices of apple.

EXTRA LEAN FACT RESEARCHERS SHOW that drinking milk helps kids maintain a healthy weight.

How to Boost Nutrition for Picky Eaters: Nobody's child eats a perfect diet. And guess what? That's okay. You can adopt a stealth approach to nutrition to get them the healthy variety of foods they need to grow and thrive. Here are some ideas:

If your child refuses milk—work around it! You know that milk is a great way for your child to get crucial body-building nutrients like calcium, potassium, magnesium, and vitamin D. Getting enough milk now means that your child is likely to have better bone density and fewer bone fractures as an adult. If she turns her nose up at milk, replace her calcium needs with other foods. Just a 4 oz serving of yogurt plus a slice of reduced fat cheddar cheese and a half cup of orange juice will meet a toddler's daily calcium needs. For older kids, try serving a piece of part-skim string cheese with a bowl of fortified oatmeal, 6 oz of low fat yogurt, and a whole grain English muffin with ¾ cup orange juice. Eggs and fish are rich in vitamin D, or you can add vitamin D supplements.

If your child likes only white bread, it's no big deal. It's true that whole wheat bread is healthier than that white bread your kids love, since whole wheat flour has more protein, fiber, and vitamin E, which combine to make your children feel fuller after a sandwich. However, only half of your child's servings of grain need to be whole. Balance out white bread by serving whole grain cereals.

If your child eats everything with ketchup, shop for the right one. Most kids love ketchup because it tastes sweet. That's because ketchup *is* sweet—every tablespoon has a teaspoon of sugar and as much salt as a handful of potato chips! Shop for brands with no sodium and those that are sweetened with regular sugar instead of high fructose corn syrup. It's worth a squirt of healthier ketchup if it means your child will eat her fish and vegetables.

EXTRA LEAN FACT IN A RECENT study, young children ate more carrots if they were served before a meal rather than during lunch.

How to Prevent Food Fights

I know from hearing my sister and my friends talk about their kids that it's easy to worry about whether your child is eating right. Whether your child seems to be a nonstop eater and looks "pudgy" to you, or your child is stick-thin and never seems to sit for more than three minutes at the dinner table, you're probably like most parents and worry about whether your child is getting enough calories and nutrients—or not enough.

The best way to know for sure is to have a straight talk with your pediatrician about your concerns. Find out your child's percentiles for height and weight and whether she's in proportion. If she is, then let it go. Most experts agree that less control is better when it comes to kids and food.

If you fight with your child about food, you don't stand a chance of winning, because your child can just eat what she wants when you're not around. You need to let your kids decide what and how much they'll eat. Again, let me emphasize that your kids will learn a lot more by watching you than by listening to you.

Instead of telling your child what to eat, show her by example. Treat food like what it is: a source of good nourishment. Present the delicious new recipes in the meal plan without making a big deal out of the number of calories or the types of nutrients your family is getting. Just enjoy eating the foods and your child most likely will, too.

If your child does seem to be constantly hungry, the portion-controlled snacks in the meal plan should help. Most kids are hungry all of the time because they're fueling up on carbohydrates like sugary cereal, bagels, noodles, and cookies, and not getting enough protein or good fats that will be digested more slowly. Try substituting yogurt or cheese sticks, both rich in protein, for those cookies and bagels, and your child will probably be more satisfied with less food.

And, if your child doesn't want to eat what you cook, don't make substitutions or go to extra work for yourself. Parents aren't short-order cooks. Make what you've planned or use the Double Duty option in the meal plan to make different meals with the same main ingredients. Cooking completely separate meals isn't just impractical and wasteful, it also destroys the family dinner dynamic you're working so hard to cultivate.

If you are serving a food that almost everyone loves, but one child hates, he can make himself a peanut butter and jelly sandwich or grab a yogurt and some fruit. There's no point in forcing a child to eat something he doesn't want. Continue to involve your child in food preparation and, bit by bit, he'll be exposed to the exciting variety of foods in the meal plan and his curiosity will eventually win out, especially if he sees the rest of you enjoying the meals.

How to Boost Your Child's Body Image: Because I work on television, I'm well aware that we live in a society where everyone on TV and in the movies looks starved, carved, and polished. Many children see movie and TV stars and think they need to look exactly like that. They start worrying about their bodies early, especially girls who absorb the message that looking good is more important than who she is. Boys aren't immune, either—the number of boys who use products like protein powders or performance supplements by the time they're in their teens is on the rise.

Sadly, children who feel bad about their bodies are more apt to eat unhealthy foods or go on unrealistic diets around puberty, at precisely the time that their bodies need a boost in nutrition to grow and develop. As a parent, the best way you can prevent your child from developing an eating disorder or being depressed about the way she looks is to help her build a positive body image. Here are a few strategies to try:

>> Emphasize healthy eating, not dieting. The fact that you're doing the *Extra Lean Family* plan is a great way to start your child down the road to good eating habits.
>> Explain the facts. Most children become self-conscious during puberty, when they may experience weight gain before getting a growth spurt. For instance, girls grow 10 inches between ages nine and sixteen, and add up to 10 pounds a year. That's normal!
>> Accept your own body image. If you're always talking about dieting and wanting to be thinner, you're sending the message that everyone's self-worth is defined by looks. Instead, show your child that it's fun to be physically active.
>> Point out the media madness. Whenever you're looking at a magazine together, point out how models are airbrushed and have teams working on their hair and makeup.

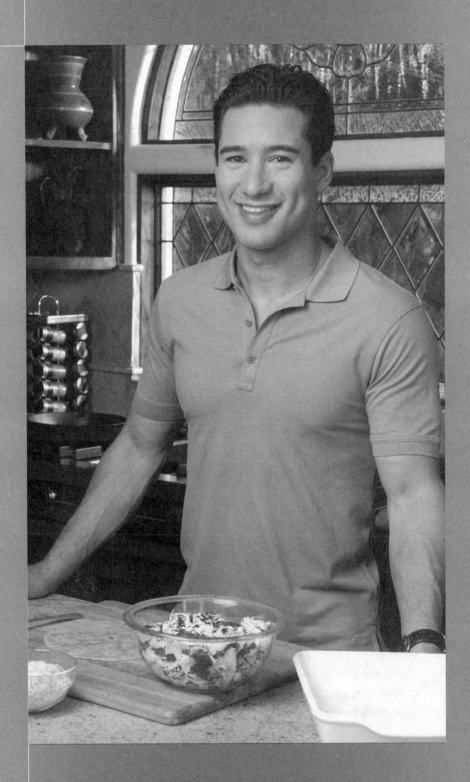

6.

other helpful tips

Active Tips to Help You and Your Family Stay *Extra Lean* and Healthy

It might seem scary to be reading this book and think, "Wow, there's so much to learn, and I'm going to have to change everything my family eats if I'm going to do it."

I assure you that while it will be a challenge, it's much easier than you think. Changing the way you eat won't happen all at once—human beings are creatures of habit, after all—but, if you approach it step-by-step, you'll see that your mind-set will gradually be altered.

Before you know it, you'll automatically start taking smaller portions, because you'll learn just how much food is the right amount for you to eat. You'll add color to your meals because you'll know that leafy greens, fruits, and vegetables are packed with nutrition—and tasty, too. You'll even have a good understanding of what the right mix of nutrients is, and you'll portion your food accordingly, using the general rule of eating ¼ protein, ¼ healthy fat, and ½ carbohydrates at each meal.

Here are tips to help you continue to build your family's awareness of what it means to live as an *Extra Lean Family*. You can use these strategies here to make quick and easy food substitutions if, say, you get stuck at a meeting after work or find yourself spending the holiday with family far from your own healthy kitchen. With just a few food and fitness tips, you can fight all of your fast-food and vending machine hunger urges.

WHEN IN DOUBT, ALWAYS REACH FOR WATER

Liquids carry sneaky calories. Beer, for instance, has 146 calories in just 12 ounces, and orange juice has 110 calories in 8 ounces. You can cut a lot of calories by switching to water or by diluting your juice, at the very least.

CHANGE UP YOUR PASTA SAUCES

We all love a creamy Alfredo sauce on our pasta, but switching to tomato sauce means that you'll save big on calories and fat. (One cup of Alfredo sauce has 360 calories and 26 fat grams, while the same amount of tomato sauce has just 75 calories and 0 fat grams.)

SNACK ON AIR-POPPED POPCORN

Few things are more fun for families than a Friday night movie at home—or even a Sunday afternoon movie if the weather is bad and you all feel like having a pajama day. Snacking on air-popped popcorn instead of oil-popped popcorn can spare your waistlines, since three cups of oil-popped popcorn has 165 calories and 9 fat grams, while the same amount of air-popped popcorn has only 40 calories and no fat at all.

DITCH REFINED CARBS

Carbohydrates are good for you. However, eating a lot of refined (highly processed) carbohydrates—things like white bread, cake, and cookies—can cause big-time sugar highs and crashes. That means that your roller coaster appetite is less likely to be satisfied. Instead, pack meals and snacks with complex carbs like fruit, beans, and vegetables.

EAT VEGETABLES FOR BREAKFAST

If the current nutrition guidelines call for your family to eat between three and five vegetable servings daily, how can you possibly fit those in? Easy: In the meal plans, you'll see that there are recipes that include veggies at breakfast!

PUT YOUR FOOD ON A PLATE

Discourage your family from grabbing food out of boxes and don't let them eat directly out of containers or bags. That makes it too tough to realize how much you're eating—you'll gobble down three servings before you know it! Put the food on a plate or in a bowl.

PICK SMART APPETIZERS

If you really want an appetizer before a meal, choosing a broth-based soup, raw vegetables, or a small salad will fill you up without adding too many calories to your main meal.

Dejunk Your Life

I define "junk food" as pretty much any food that is high in calories, fat, and/or sugar without delivering any nutrition. We see junk food in abundance everywhere in our culture: in our supermarkets and restaurants, on TV, and in the movie theaters. No wonder our kids are junk food addicts, especially if we have tendencies in that direction ourselves!

I certainly indulge in junk food now and then, especially on the weekends or after a big workout. While it's fine to eat a treat now and then, the problem with junk foods is that they just leave us feeling unsatisfied while basically delivering all sorts of empty, or even unhealthy, calories. Junking your family's junk food addiction should be easier once everyone gets on track and starts following the meal plan, because you'll all be eating lots of frequent, small meals with the right balance of protein, carbs, and fat.

As you start the plan, it may be tempting to cheat with junk food snacks, especially for kids who are on their own during part of the day, or for you and your spouse at work or on the commute home. Weekends are also big junk food days for most people, because we're on the go to sports practices or movies or parties.

How can your family junk their junk food addiction? Here are a few tips to make it easier:

Identify the time of day that each of you is most likely to cave into a junk food craving. For you, it might be that 10 a.m. post-breakfast time, while your kids may be craving junk food after school or before bed because that's what they're used to. Be especially prepared with healthy alternatives for those times, or even schedule activities then.

Always choose food and beverages that offer nutrients as well as calories. For instance, a can of soda a day can lead to a 15-pound weight gain in just one year, and you get no nutrients in return!

Avoid any food that has a high sugar content, partially hydrogenated oils, or high fructose corn syrup in the ingredients list.

Keep healthy alternatives in sight—like apples on the counter instead of a cookie jar.

If you need something crunchy, put seedless grapes in a bowl instead of chips.

Focus on the first few bites. Your taste buds may be satisfied after just ten bites—and maybe that's all you need. Just wait ten minutes before you start eating again.

Leave food on your plate. It's really okay. Nobody will yell at you. Don't eat more than you need to stop feeling hungry.

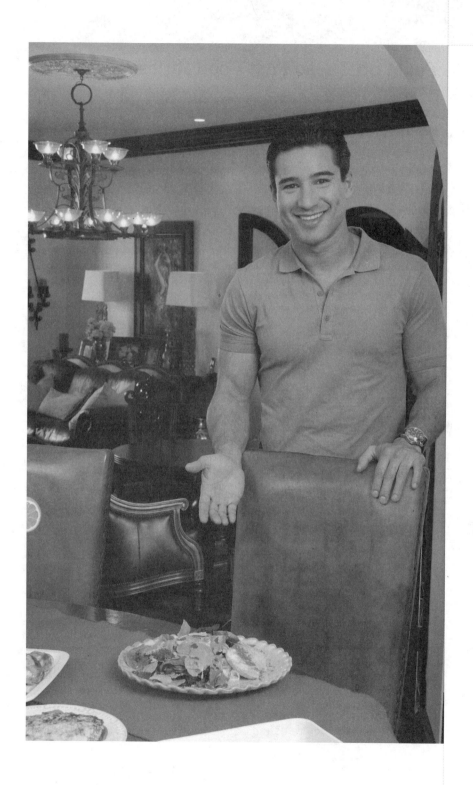

Feast on These Fast Food Rules

Let's face it: there are going to be times when you and your kids are on the road after music lessons or basketball practice, you haven't made it to the grocery store, and you're going to need to feed the starving hordes. The good news is that you're still eating as a family, and you can now get relatively nutritious meals at most fast-food chains. Ideally, you'll still follow that 50 percent carbs, 25 percent protein, 25 percent fats balance, but the food choices here are really more important than the micronutrients if you want to keep down the calories, harmful fats, sugar, and salt your family is consuming. Just follow these rules when you order:

>> Know what you're eating. Before you're caught up short waiting in a drive-through line, log onto calorieking.com, a Web site that offers nutritional information for most fast-food restaurants.

>> Forget salty meats. Bacon and sausage are high in salt and saturated fats.

>> Skip the soda. Fountain drinks are loaded with sugar and calories, and they come in buckets rather than cups at most fast-food chains. Stick to water or take advantage of the low fat milk most places offer.

>> Pass on the salad dressing. Nothing ups the calories more on a salad than the high-cal dressings that come in those packets. Use a tiny bit of dressing, or opt for the low fat or fat-free dressing if the chain has it on hand.

>> Order child-size portions. Most child-size portions have fewer calories and fat.

>> Swap mayo for mustard. Even supposedly healthy grilled chicken sandwiches are slathered in high-calorie mayonnaise or other sauces. Plain mustard is a healthier option on everything.

>> Cut back on cheese. Most pizza places will put half the usual amount if you ask ahead of time, and eliminating the cheese on sandwiches can save you a bundle of calories and decrease the saturated fat you're eating.

Fool Your Appetite

You may think that you have no control over your appetite—or yourself—because you keep eating a second helping of food when you shouldn't, or even polishing off a bag of fries on your way home from work. There are lots of tricks you can use to outwit your appetite, such as:

>> Use smaller size serving spoons, plates, and glasses. Research shows that people eat more if they have big bowls, glasses, and utensils, because the temptation is to fill them. Try using a salad plate instead of a dinner plate to fool your eye, and use soup spoons instead of serving spoons to dole out food.

>> Don't do anything else when you eat. Most people overeat if they have a meal or a snack while driving, reading, or watching TV. Always find a place to sit and eat without distractions, and put your utensils down between bites to slow yourself down. That will help you recognize when you're full. Or, if you can't avoid eating while doing something else, portion out your food and don't go back for seconds.

>> Keep food out of sight at work. If your coworker always has a bowl of candy on her desk, you know how hard it is to resist, right? The same is true at home. Keep food out of sight so that you're less tempted to eat when you shouldn't.

>> Order first in a restaurant. It's tempting to order an appetizer if all of your friends are getting them. Try to place your order first, so that you get exactly what you should eat, and not what your friends are eating.

>> Get more sleep. Tired people make bad food choices.

>> Drink your wine with your meal, not before. Otherwise you'll be more tempted to have a second glass.

Make Family Fitness Part of Your *Extra Lean Family* Plan

I can't possibly talk about eating *Extra Lean* as a family without also talking to you about physical activity. Healthy fitness and healthy foods go together to create a lifestyle that's more energetic and productive for everyone. Yet, we're raising our children in a world where the speed of technology, which has made our lives so much more efficient and fast-paced, has slowed us down physically. That inactivity is killing us.

Take control of the iPods, TVs, and computers in your house. Make physical fitness a priority for your children. Sign them up for sports teams, at least one a season, if you can. The daily commitment that kids learn from coaches and other teammates is something that will stay with them their entire lives. For me, the values I learned on the wrestling mat in high school, like dedication and determination, are values I still practice today.

I know as well as anyone that there are only a certain number of hours in a day, and that you can probably find ways right now to fill every single second of every single minute. Making strides to overhaul your daily routines so that you can make room for family fitness is just as daunting as changing the way you eat. If you work long hours already, and the kids are involved in school and activities, where does that free time come from for family fitness?

Walking is a great way to start exercising more as a family. It takes no special skills, ability, or equipment, and everyone can do it together. It's also a great way to keep up those family conversations you've got going at the dinner table.

Whatever is holding your family back from being more active, I want you to take a minute to consider the reasons below that most people give for not getting up off the couch or away from the computer to move around. I'm betting that one of these reasons is yours—and that I can help you overcome that self-imposed obstacle.

Reason #1: I don't have enough time to be active. The reason most people give for not exercising is that they're short on time during the day. I completely understand that perception, but I also know that's exactly what it is: a perception, and not the truth. How many things in life do you give priority to that could be replaced by exercise? For instance, how many minutes a day do you spend on your cell phone or surfing the Web?

One thing I've learned is that it doesn't take hours a day to get more fit. Even if you spend just a few minutes every day doing some body weight exercises in your home, or walk on the treadmill while watching TV, you can burn excess fat and extra calories. You'll also be setting a great example for your kids. They may be active already if they're involved in sports, but they'll remember seeing you working out, and that will make them more likely to join you now or to do the same when they get older.

WHAT THE RESEARCH SAYS ABOUT
physical **fitness**

Kids are slowing down. The National Institutes of Health reports that nearly one-third of our schools' students are not getting the minimum hour of exercise daily that's considered essential.

Fitter bodies = faster minds. Children who scored low on a standardized physical fitness assessment tool also ranked further down the scale on state achievement tests than kids who scored high in fitness, according to researchers.

Inactivity leads to more than just weight gain. Research shows that people who are inactive not only gain weight, but are also more susceptible to health problems such as heart disease and diabetes.

Reason #2: I can't get motivated because nothing I do makes a difference in how I look. Rome wasn't built in a day. You can't expect yourself to completely transform your body overnight. Just as you're doing with the *Extra Lean Family* plan to eat a healthier, more varied diet, you can take small steps to achieve reasonable goals on a regular basis. Walk around the block as a family after dinner. Ride bikes together twice a week. You don't have to run a marathon or swim the English Channel. Just think in terms of getting active for at least half an hour a day and breaking a sweat if possible.

Reason #3: Exercise is boring. The key to starting to exercise and, more importantly, to sticking with it, is to find something you enjoy doing. Make it a priority for your family to explore different activities, and let your kids choose some of the things you try. You won't know that you love tennis or hiking unless you try it. The kids might just choose tossing a ball in the backyard, but that's fine. Anything that gets everyone out of the house and moving around is a good thing.

Boost Your Energy and Metabolism with Pre- and Post-Workout Nutrition

Just like you, I have trouble fitting in my exercise most days between work, household, and family responsibilities. No matter how busy I am, though, I make time for workouts. My goal is to sweat a little more every day. I just don't always know, from one day to the next, when I'll be free to hit the gym, go running, swim, dance, or do any of my other favorite activities.

My unpredictable schedule, together with my commitment to staying active, means that it's important for me to stay fueled with the right healthy foods all day long, since I'll never know exactly when my next window of opportunity will present itself and I can grab some workout time.

Maybe you do have a consistent workout schedule—let's say you always hit the gym right before work, or always take a walk at lunchtime. If that's the case, be very certain to plan your meals and snacks accordingly. If you have a good idea about what time you'll be going for your run or hitting that exercise class, make sure you have your snacks (both pre- and post-workout) handy, so that you can fuel up and replenish with perfect timing. The better you are at creating those habits, the more successful you'll be at getting into shape and staying that way.

If your schedule is as unpredictable as mine, just be sure to have those healthy snacks at hand when you need them for your pre- and post-workout fuel. Whether you're a dad who likes to join pickup basketball games a couple of times a week, a teenager on a hockey team, or a mom who tries to make it to Zumba or Pilates a couple of nights each week, eating right before and right after your workouts is key both to keeping your metabolism geared to working efficiently and to putting in your best performance on the field, dance floor, or court.

Personally, I like to fuel up on both carbohydrates and a good supply of protein both before and after a workout. When it comes to my pre-workout fuel, I don't like to feel too full, nor do I like to feel hungry. I go for foods that will sustain me without weighing me down. About half an hour before a training session, my favorite food choices tend to be slow-digesting carbs (the kind that are jam-packed with fuel and that will stay within my system the longest), like oatmeal, fruit, or whole-grain bread.

I'll also add in some protein both before and after a workout session, because protein is used by your body to build blocks of lean tissue. Experts also agree that eating enough protein can help lessen the onset of muscle soreness for most athletes. In other words, eating right can really help you recover from your workout as well as pump you up for exercise.

The thing I like to eat least before heading to a workout are those quick-digesting carbs like sugary foods or sports drinks. Your body doesn't get a lot out of those during a session, so I save those for after I'm finished working out to help replenish my system quickly. Solid pre- and post-workout nutrition isn't just for adults, of course. What your children eat both before and after athletic practices at school, a pickup game of soccer with friends, or even a game of tag in the neighborhood, will go a long way toward increasing their stamina while they play. And that stamina, in turn, will make them better performers and happier players, so that they'll be more inclined to keep being active while also establishing good eating habits.

With younger children, just keep the basic principles—slow carbohydrates and protein before playing, simple carbohydrates and protein afterward—in mind, plus lots of water. Forget fast food on the way to the practice field. Instead, hand your kids a high-fiber granola bar, a piece of fruit, and a glass of milk before the game. Then, when they come back home, make them a fruit smoothie or let them have Gatorade.

High school kids should always eat a snack before sports practices. I can't imagine having to go through an entire football or wrestling practice on an empty stomach. Not only is it uncomfortable feeling hungry while trying to play sports, but it will without a doubt hurt your child's performance on the field or on the court. You can't perform athletically at your best if you have practice at four o'clock but you ate lunch at eleven thirty. If your child can sneak in a snack at two or three o'clock, practice will be that much more enjoyable and productive.

After practice, it will probably be right around dinnertime, so in many cases that can serve as an adequate post-practice meal. But, if your child is really hungry and dinner won't be served for another hour or so, feel free to let him or her have a small nutritious snack to replenish the nutrients lost while practicing.

The following are the best carbs for both your pre- and post-workout:

GREAT PRE-WORKOUT CARBOHYDRATES

These carbs power me through my workouts. Slow-digesting carbohydrates like these keep insulin levels down during training as well, helping you burn more fat for fuel during rest periods.

Bananas
Oranges
Apples
Oatmeal
Granola
Sweet potatoes
Raisins
Whole wheat bread

GO FOR THESE POST-WORKOUT CARBOHYDRATES

After a workout is actually the safest time to eat fast-digesting carbs without worrying about storing them as fat, so I add small amounts of these kinds of carbs to my other slow-digesting kinds. Enjoy these ONLY after rigorous exercise.

Gatorade
Angel food cake
Sorbet
White bread
Grits
Cream of wheat

MORE ON WORKOUT NUTRITION

You and your family need to fuel your bodies for exercise. Here are some more useful tips for what to eat and drink before, during, and after a workout:

An hour before you go to the gym or get on the playing field, fuel up on healthy carbohydrates for energy. Eating too much protein can make you feel heavy and sluggish because it's harder for your body to convert protein to energy.

Half an hour before your workout, a cup of yogurt can give you a quick, light protein boost.

If you have only ten minutes before hitting the gym, choose some healthy veggie chips to snack on for a quick boost.

During your workout, drink plain or flavored water. But, if you and your children are really exerting yourselves or it's an incredibly hot day, grab a sports drink.

Right after your workout, you're going to want to go for healthy carbs again—even fruit juice. Post-workout foods should definitely contain protein and can be a simple snack—even chocolate milk has a nice balance of carbs, protein, and fluid. Follow up a post-workout snack with a more substantial meal within two to three hours. Then it's the time for a "meal" with a healthy balance of carbs, protein, and fats.

Holidays & Special Occasions

Holidays are tricky when it comes to healthy eating. There's so much great food on the table that you don't usually get other times of the year. Plus, everyone is encouraging you to have another helping of mashed potatoes with gravy, or try this pie, or why not have a piece of both pies? Everyone is in the spirit of the holiday and healthy eating takes a backseat to the celebration.

With luck, by the time a holiday rolls around, your family will have already used the *Extra Lean Family* plan to build everyone's awareness of what it means to eat the right amounts of nutritious food in a way that will give each of you vital energy and keep you all in good health. You'll already know what healthy portions look like and how to balance your intake of nutrients, and ideally you've already put a family fitness plan in place that's keeping you all moving.

It's temping to toss out every good intention with the holidays. Your schedule is hectic, you have family visiting or you're traveling, or you might say to yourselves that Thanksgiving or Easter or Hanukkah comes but once a year, and give in to that third helping of dinner, plus two desserts. However, there are some great strategies for healthy holiday eating that I've learned along the way. These strategies can help you and your family celebrate while still maintaining some control over what you eat, so that you can spare yourselves the discomfort of having binged and eaten unhealthy foods despite your goals.

Here are a few things I do to get myself through these special days with the most enjoyment and the least backtracking on my *Extra Lean* goals:

>> Make a game plan before the holiday. Picture what you're going to eat before the big day.
>> Exercise that morning if possible.
>> Manage your stress. Get extra sleep, read a good book, walk the dog: do whatever it takes to put yourself in a calm frame of mind for the holiday, because stress is often a trigger for eating comforting, rich foods.

>> Eat fruit and a protein-rich snack before dinner, or before going to parties, to avoid the temptation of arriving at a holiday dinner hungry and ready to overeat.

>> If you're not cooking the meal, ask the host if you can bring a dish, and make it an *Extra Lean* dish.

>> Drink plenty of water to help control your appetite—you'll feel fuller faster, and you'll be less tempted by alcohol and soda served at the holiday party.

>> Avoid appetizers and other finger foods. These are often rich in calories.

>> Choose white meat turkey and remove the skin—this has half the calories of the darker meat with the skin left on.

>> When you fill your plate, keep portions in mind, and follow the 50 percent protein, 25 percent fat, 25 percent carbohydrates rule.

>> Eat slowly—remember that it takes up to twenty minutes before your brain can register that you're feeling full.

>> Politely decline seconds.

>> Avoid gravy and foods made with heavy sauces.

>> If you drink wine, mix carbonated water into it—wine spritzers have fewer calories.

>> Allow yourself to have a small piece of your favorite dessert, and savor every bite.

>> Start a new tradition: Convince everyone to take a family walk after dinner!

With this book, you have the tools to help you make healthy choices. You are now part of an *Extra Lean Family*. You understand what that means now, and you're prepared to maintain your new approach to food, so that you and your family can look and feel healthy while eating all the foods you love.

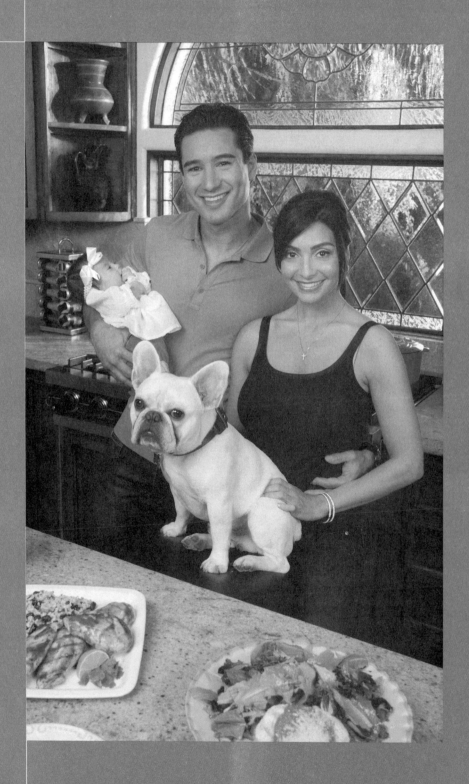

conclusion

EXTRA LEAN FAMILY provides a detailed look into how my family and I approach food and how we eat. Good health and long-lasting happiness starts right in the kitchen, where you and your family can discover a variety of foods that will boost your metabolisms. I wrote this book so that you and your family can learn to love food and live longer, more energetic, and productive lives—together.

To successfully change the way you eat so that your metabolism will work for you in the long run, follow these key principles:

Understand the *Extra Lean* principles of balancing the vital macronutrients, practicing portion control, and eating frequently to unleash the metabolism's optimal efficiency. Once you know how to make your metabolism work for you, seek out a variety of vegetables, fruits, whole grains, lean meat and fish, and healthy oils and nuts that will help you burn fat and keep the weight off. Then, test your knowledge of balancing these foods in the right amounts by practicing what a healthy plate looks like. If you and your family can remember how much you need to eat to boost your metabolisms, then this is the only nutritional foundation you'll ever need to continue losing weight.

Prepare your family for *Extra Lean* living by evaluating the foods you eat to determine what should stay in the kitchen and what should be tossed. Just as crucial is learning to navigate your way through the grocery store so that you don't pick up or revert to previous eating habits. It's these types of tangible actions that will keep your mind focused on staying healthy and strong.

Maintain your family's nutritional foundation when everyday life happens by staying focused. Understand why every meal matters and which foods are best for your body and metabolism during the different times of the day. Plan meals ahead by using the prep highlights featured in the meal plans and use the Double Duty Options to satisfy all of the people in your household. Remember, good food should not be sacrificed because of lack of time and a busy house.

Finally, experience *Extra Lean* living every day by following the way the meals have been set up and prepared in the plan. As I've learned by educating myself, and through my own trial-and-error experiments in cooking, there are lots of quick, easy, and less expensive alternatives for feeding your family that are much healthier than buying packaged convenience foods or eating out. The meals in this book contain a balance of 50 percent carbs, 25 percent protein, and 25 percent fat; offer a variety of delicious foods that will keep your family satisfied; and can be cooked in twenty minutes or less. All of these important factors will help you and your family enjoy cooking good food in your kitchen for life.

Remember, your children are watching what you eat, probably as closely as you're watching them. Ensure their health comes first each and every day by making good food the focus and help them live a more fulfilling life, the kind of life that can be enjoyed by having the right attitude toward food.

If the thought of family meals has new meaning for you after reading this book, then I will have done my job. If you agree that food is fuel that can be enjoyed and cherished by anyone under your roof, then I can write these sentences with pride.

While I'm humbled and inspired by your willingness to take back your health, you, too, should be filled with joy and hope. The better able you are to learn and educate your family about the importance of sensible eating, the longer and more abundant life each and every person sitting around your table stands to live. That's the key: being willing to stand up and make the commitment to make a change in your lives together.

My inspiration comes from both my passion for food and health and my duty to make sure that everyone I love the most lives a happy and healthy life. Growing up with my mom's homemade cooking and eating meals with my family taught me to love food, which is the most solid foundation for my health right now.

Always remember that loving food through family meals will allow you and your family to live healthy, happy, and *Extra Lean* for life.

acknowledgments

My publisher Raymond Garcia, editor Kim Suarez, and everyone at Penguin: Thank you for your continued confidence and partnership.

Dana Angelo White: Again, your nutritional advice and delicious recipes grace these pages. Thank you for all you do.

Holly Robinson: Thank you for your invaluable contributions. Astounding work.

Mark Schulman, my manager: You set the standard for excellence.

Diana Sillero, my assistant: Nobody keeps me on track like you do.

index